Live, Love and Thrive with Herpes

A Holistic Guide For Women

By

DR. KELLY MARTIN SCHUH

© 2012 www.PinkTent.com

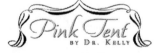

Illustrations by Katherine Homes and Megan Yalkut/hamsadesign.com

Medical Disclaimer: This material is for educational purposes only and is not intended as diagnosis, treatment, or prescription for any disease. This is not a replacement for medical care. Your health-care provider must always review any changes in prescriptions, diet, supplements, or natural remedies first.

I dedicate this book to my husband, Richard, for believing in me more than I believed in myself. Thank you for your unwavering love and support.

May this book uplift the millions of women around the world who have been screaming in silence.

Table of Contents

CHAPTER 1: HOW I GOT HERPES: AN OUTWARD JOURNEY TURNS INWARD..... 1

Medicine: A Passion from Childhood 4

Herpes in the Himalayas 7

My First Herpes Outbreak.. 18

CHAPTER 2: A HOLISTIC APPROACH: LOOKING AT HEALTH AND HERPES
FROM A WHOLE PERSPECTIVE... 21

Signposts, Not Symptoms.. 24

A Healing Crisis: Are Your Symptoms Getting Worse?.................... 26

The Impact of Our Emotions on Symptoms.............................. 27

Is There a Magic Bullet For Herpes?... 28

Eastern and Western Perspectives on "Healing" Herpes 30

Herpes "Cures" – Is the FDA Really Protecting Us?...................... 34

Consciously Implementing Change: Lianna's Story...................... 36

CHAPTER 3: THE ROLE OF GRIEF AND THE POWER OF FORGIVENESS
IN MANAGING YOUR HERPES 39

Flowing with Grief: Integrating Your Emotions 40

Get it OUT of Your System! Share your story! 44

The Act of Forgiveness 45

Forgiveness Is The Gift You Give Yourself................................. 46

Forgiving the Unforgivable 48

An Exercise of Forgiveness 50

CHAPTER 4: CULTIVATING A HEALING PERSPECTIVE, INTUITION
AND CHAKRA HEALING 53

A Learner In Action.. 54

Victim And Victor 57

Drink the Juice of Positive Thinking 58

You Can Heal Your Life – Louise Hay's Story.............................. 60

Begin to Cancel Out Negative Self Talk With Positive Declarations 62

Being In The Flow 64

Using Intuition to Heal Your Herpes 65

Forms of Intuition... 66

The Elevator Exercise: Getting Out of Your Head and into Your Body . 70

Healing Herpes Through Your Chakras 71

First Chakra Clearing Exercise: Your Grounding Cord 73
Revitalizing Chakra Three: Call Your Power Back! 74
Healing Chakras One-Four: Breath is Life................................. 75

CHAPTER 5: HERPES FAQ AND FACTS ABOUT PREGNANCY 79
The Truth Revealed: Questions and Answers 79
Q & A on Testing... 96
Questions About Diagnosis 99
Q & A on Herpes and Partners 102
Herpes and Pregnancy: What Are the True Risks to the Newborn?....113

CHAPTER 6: HIDDEN TRIGGERS AND TOXICITIES 123
The Toxic Umbrella: Heavy Metal and Chemical Toxicity 123
Toxic Food And Why We Need To Supplement 124
A Common Mineral Imbalance 126
Cosmetics and Personal Care...127
Electromagnetic Pollution 129
There's Something Fishy Going On 130
Identifying and Removing Toxins From Your Life 132
A Solution To The Toxic Umbrella 134
The Top 10 Hidden Herpes Triggers Your Doctor Never Told You......136
Food: Know Your Peas and Carrots...139
Lysine and Arginine 142
Frequent Outbreaks? Omit The Nightshades 144
Shopping Guidelines Summary 144

CHAPTER 7: SOLUTIONS: SELF CARE PLAN, SUPPLEMENTS AND
HEALING REMEDIES 147
Quick Start Self Care Plan..148
Herpes Self Assessment: Your Unique Imbalances 151
Supplements and Herbs 154
Healing Remedies 156
Specific Remedies For Oral Herpes 163

CHAPTER 8: LEARNING TO LOVE YOURSELF AND OTHERS 165
We Are Gems 165
Are You Open To Love? 168
Feeling Sexy And Deserving Of Love 170
My First "Talk" After Diagnosis..171
Practice Makes Perfect 172

The Fear Of Rejection 173

Why Waiting to Have "the Talk" is Not the Best Idea 174

When would YOU Want to Be Told ? 175

The Do's and the Don'ts 176

Taking the Charge Out of Your Story 181

Eliminating Your Fears Before Having "the Talk" 183

In Parting 186

Beneath The Pink Tent 187

Healing Tools and Resources- A Bonus Section 189

Appendix A: Exercises and Meditations 189

Appendix B: Dr. Kelly's Guide to Healing Modalities 199

Appendix C: Additional Resources 211

References 215

Index 217

Live, Love and Thrive with Herpes
A Holistic Guide for Women

INTRODUCTION

I have lived with herpes for fourteen years. At several points along the way, I questioned my ability to heal and to discover partnership. I thought that I would never be able to deliver a healthy baby naturally. Herpes presented me with the greatest challenge of self-discovery that I have ever faced. I wrote this book because I believe that in rising to meet this challenge, I have gained knowledge, perspective, and practices that can help and empower every woman with herpes.

No matter what anyone tells you, you are a beautiful, courageous woman. How do I know this? Because you have picked up this book, and you are looking to live a life different than your current reality. You are looking for answers that will enable you to live, love, and thrive, despite having herpes.

If you are depressed, confused, ashamed, grieving, feeling like a leper, and screaming in silence, welcome to the world of herpes in our culture—one that has no qualms about placing half-naked women in prominent media situations and yet would never consider talking about the facts of sex or the truth about herpes. Since herpes is a sexually transmitted infection, the topic is a magnet for jokes, scams, and myths.

So, why am I revealing the truth about herpes and teaching women how to live vibrant, healthy lives with it? First and foremost, women are three to four times more likely to get herpes than men. I have also met many women with herpes who have a history of sexual abuse. This is a double whammy of shame, and an affront to our self-confidence as sexual beings. This leads many to a life of despair and self-imprisoned celibacy.

If we are not celibate, our doctors also tell us that we might never be able to bear children naturally. This was the greatest blow to me when I discovered, at twenty-three, that I had herpes. Who would ever love me and my "damaged goods"? I thought.

The solution? Women, by nature, support and uplift one another when we are able to reveal our deepest, darkest secrets. So, allow me to stand in my power so that you can stand in yours. I too continue to grow as a leader in this bold endeavor, to share my personal story about herpes and expose the truth. In teaching you how to naturally manage herpes, you can become stronger, healthier, more loving, and more radiant than ever. I am willing to place my heart and reputation on the line, knowing that my vulnerability could bring you strength. I have nothing to be ashamed of in regards to my herpes status.

By putting this information out into the public eye, I intend to shed a bright light on this dark and often frightening diagnosis. There are many faces to herpes: old, young, rich, poor, educated, illiterate, promiscuous, and even abstinent. Yes, abstinent! It is my mission to de-stigmatize herpes and reveal the truth about a virus that affects upward of 80 to 90 percent of the American population, in some form or another. More shocking and disturbing than that is that 85 percent of people who have genital herpes don't even know they have it!

If you do not learn how to love again, as this book will teach you, then you will not be able to experience the gifts life has in store for you. Through shame I learned compassion, through fear I found true love, and through turmoil I learned peace. I was able to find love, marry, and give birth to the most precious gift of all, a healthy baby girl. I did this all naturally in the privacy of our own home. I would have never thought these dreams could come to fruition for me.

Herpes makes you feel like you are on the bleachers while everyone else is out on the dance floor, much like the typical, awkward teen dance. Please hold onto your faith and take this chance to dance. For when herpes closes one door, another one opens, one filled with personal growth, exploration, love, and better health. To give and receive love is the ultimate human experience. Don't allow herpes to withhold your love, for the world needs your love, courage, and self-acceptance. Become the learner, for you have an excellent opportunity at totally altering your path in life.

Included in the following pages is a capsule summary of the chapters to follow. Give yourself the time you need to integrate this material. If your heart feels heavy and your breath shallow, stop, breathe, and regroup. This is an excellent time to do one of the meditations or exercises found in the bonus section of the book. You can think of each of the chapters as mini-books and gravitate to the areas that interest you most, absorbing, reflecting, and practicing step by step along the way. This is a book you will reference on many occasions. It is meant to be a complete guide for your whole journey.

I humbly hope that in distilling what I've learned the hard way about living with herpes, I've made your journey a few steps lighter.

May you share love, seek peace, inspire hope, and scatter joy.

Live. Love. Thrive
Dr. Kelly Martin Schuh, D.C.

Summary of Chapters

How I Got Herpes: An Outward Journey Turns Inward

This section reveals how I contracted the herpes virus 14 years ago, while searching for my life purpose. Although we each have a unique story to tell, we can all connect and relate to the initial shock and devastation that a herpes diagnosis evokes.

A Holistic Approach: Looking at Health and Herpes from a Whole Perspective

Learning to look at your spiritual, mental, and physical selves as a whole process develops a critical perspective that has helped me greatly over the years. I'll share how my perspectives have morphed over the years and how I came to adopt a truly holistic approach to healing herpes. I will teach you a few ways you can start applying positive practices from all three of these intertwined spheres to live — and feel — better.

The Role of Grief and The Power of Forgiveness in Managing Your Herpes

Contracting herpes can leave too many women feeling depressed, betrayed, angry, and resentful. Learn how consciously approaching the critical processes of grief and forgiveness is central to your healing process and to set you free.

Cultivating A Healing Perspective, Intuition and Chakra Healing

The mind and body are powerful healers, and when they are in synch with one another, miracles can occur. I'll introduce you to your inner guru and teach you some techniques that are invaluable in confronting your health issues, reprogramming your self-sabotaging thoughts, and getting in tune with the natural energies that help your body heal.

Herpes FAQ And Facts About Pregnancy

There's a lot of misinformation and myth floating around out there. This section will give you the facts about herpes, partnerships, and pregnancy, creating a solid foundation for yourself and those you care about.

Hidden Triggers and Toxicities

How we eat and the substances we expose ourselves to have an enormous impact on outbreaks. In this section, I give you some practical tips for managing your diet and personal environment to minimize outbreaks and feel your best.

Solutions: Self-Care Plan, Supplements and Healing Remedies

This section is a practical, Quick Start Self-Care Plan to turn fear into action and a no-nonsense plan for living day to day with herpes. You'll learn what supplements to take and how to manage your symptoms all naturally.

Learning to Love Yourself and Others

Many feel as though herpes is the end of their ability to love. Managed with care and consciousness, it's just the beginning. I'll show you how to overcome your fears of having "the Talk" and will guide you through this intimate discussion about your herpes status.

Healing Tools and Resources – A Bonus Section

This section will nourish your soul and integrate your emotions. Dive into these exercises. Discover new healing modalities and resources you can explore as your curiosity and inspiration dictate.

ONE

How I Got Herpes: An Outward Journey Turns Inward

[S]he who knows others is wise;
[s]he who knows [herself] is enlightened.

—LAO-TZU

Below are two excerpts from my 1998 journal, when I contracted herpes on a post-college trip to the Himalayas.

Kathmandu—January 2, 1998

Yesterday was one of the worst days of my life. The doctor in the clinic thinks that Kevin gave me herpes. We spent the whole day trying to get to the clinic. It's Visit Nepal 98, and yesterday was their huge festival.

The doctor gave me some cream and medicine, which I am to take five times a day. I'm plagued by great sadness, feelings of guilt, embarrassment, and stupidity.

How could I have been so damned weak and stupid? If I had not been so lonely and if I had listened to my instincts about Kevin's lip, this would have never happened! If this is herpes, I'll have to deal with it for the rest of my life. It could even be passed on to my children. Supposedly, I won't even be able to have a vaginal delivery; I'll have to have a C-section.

Last night I went straight home from the clinic and cried myself in and out of sleep from five p.m. until nine a.m. I feel so dirty and gross, like I've done something terrible and I'm being punished for it. I keep hoping it's bacterial or something else. Only an antibody test can confirm the diagnosis. Kevin came to my room last night, and I couldn't even look at him. I don't know whom to turn to or what to do. I even considered ending my trip. Everything has changed for me! I guess I'll try and cope and continue onward. Maybe I can be tested prior to returning home, so I know what I'm dealing with. If only I could talk to friends and family in person. I keep hoping that I've been ill informed. Maybe I got this strange thing from the hot springs, or possibly the sore on Kevin's lip isn't herpes. I'll keep my fingers crossed, but I'll assume the worst. What a horrible new year! I cried as the clock struck midnight. I'm disgusted with myself and hope that the damage is repairable.

Kathmandu—January 6, 1998

I have seen two doctors now and have all the info that I need for now. It is herpes!!!! I can't believe that of all the things that could have happened to me, out of all the things I've been informed about and careful of, I am stuck with a venereal disease. I feel so stupid. I will not let this disease ruin my life. I do not deserve this and have been so very careful all of my life. No one ever told me that oral herpes was so dangerous and contagious. Our health educational system is to blame. A long road of self-discovery and healing awaits me. I must learn from this and turn this horrible fate into something positive.

I will allow myself to feel the pain, hurt, guilt, sorrow, and everything else. It is the natural way to heal. Baby steps. One day at a time. Life can come and slam you on your ass when you're not looking. It's when you're so worried about the major problems and hazards in life that you forget to look at what's waiting in the wings. That which is often so evident is somehow hidden. As Peter explained, "You hit the road to learn what real life is all about." This is true. Life is hard sometimes, and there are difficult lessons to learn. I could have died in an avalanche at Annapurna Base Camp, but God spared me that. I could have been born into poverty or live in Algeria where four hundred people were just massacred and mutilated. Life is unfair and I have been unlucky. The question that awaits me now is, what's next?

Medicine: A Passion from Childhood

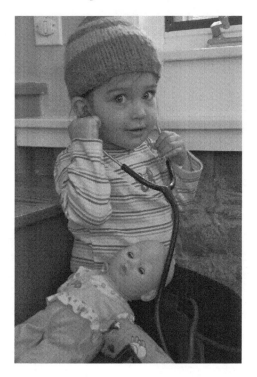

From a very young age, I can remember donning my mother's crisp, white nursing cap and playing doctor with my friends. I had a keen interest in the human body and how it functioned. I loved the sleuthing aspect of deciphering a most probable "diagnosis" from a list of symptoms and then "prescribing" a solution for what ailed my playtime patients. Most of the care plans back then were centered on a bowl of chicken noodle soup, a big hug, and a prescription to keep my patients healthy. When asked, "What do you want to be when you grow up?" my answer was always the same. I wanted to be a doctor. My instincts pulled me toward the field of helping others heal. I couldn't have known back then where that course would ultimately take me. I couldn't possibly know that my desire for world travel and adventure would inescapably lead back into myself.

I was fortunate to have spent my childhood in a loving home in Wilmington, Delaware, with my mother, father, and sister, Michelle, who was five years my senior. Mom and Dad grew up within a few blocks of each other. They met at an ice cream social, arranged by my grandparents when Mom was a sophomore in high school. Dad was a shy, introverted jazz musician, a freshman music major at West Chester University in Pennsylvania. They fell in love, married, and raised my sister and me within miles of their childhood homes. They still live there, where they recently celebrated their forty-third wedding anniversary.

My introduction to medicine and teaching was through my mother, who had graduated at the top of her nursing class. I admired her for her intellect and nurturing bedside manner. Doctors loved her for her skill in briefing them on patient management and course of treatment, although she didn't want me to waste my time cleaning bedpans and taking orders from doctors. She wanted *me* to become a doctor. She wanted me to shoot for the stars and not to settle for anything else.

My mom felt that for her, a doctor's career was out of reach. She was a young, Christian woman from a strictly traditional, middle-class upbringing. My grandmother's idea of education began and ended with the Ten Commandments. At the age of twelve, Grandmom had to quit her studies at a one-room schoolhouse to help tend the fields in Felton, Delaware. In those times, the mark of a strong woman was being able to make a mean casserole, keep a tidy house, and raise the kids.

From the time I was five years old, I loved tagging along with my mother. I was constantly found by her side as she taught advanced CPR to other nurses at the American Heart Association. I was her shadow, although she called me her Little Miss Sunshine. From ceramics to crocheting, my mother created space for me with kid-sized projects that allowed me to follow along with her creative endeavors. We were inseparable, at least up until three p.m., on the days when she would have to work the evening shift in the Pediatric ICU of the local hospital. My father, then an elementary school music teacher with a striking resemblance to Fred Rogers from *Mr. Rogers' Neighborhood*, would rush home from work to watch my sister and me. The aromas of crockpot meals filled the air. Late each night, my father would wrap us up in blankets and load us up in our old station wagon to pick Mom up from work.

I gravitated hungrily toward both academics and sports as an adolescent. During this time, medicine still fascinated me: while my friends followed *Beverly Hills 90210*, I would watch *ER* with my mom so we could discuss the symptoms and diagnoses the doctors gave. While that fascination remained steadfast, I vacillated as to whether or not I wanted to commit to the grueling work of becoming a physician. It wasn't the academic challenge that intimidated me—it was the fear of living the stressful, passionless, unhappy existence that seemed to define so many physicians.

I had years of experience through my early twenties as a candy striper—a nonmedical volunteer—in a local emergency room. I continued on as a medical assistant, searching for the specialty that would best suit me. I dabbled in orthopedics, pediatrics, the ER, internal medicine, and women's health. In all those years of volunteering and working, I never met any doctor who was truly passionate about his or her chosen profession and the life doctors were living. It seemed like doctors' life force—or *prana*, as the ancients called it—had been zapped right out of their souls. They all complained of malpractice lawsuits, pressure from insurance companies, time constraints, escalating paperwork, agonizing documentation, and the challenges of providing excellent patient care.

The bottom line for me was that most medical doctors I had met were miserable. Most were stressed out, undernourished, and overweight. Their initial intention of making a difference in the world was replaced by the grim, primal drive to just make it through the day. Patients were no longer at the heart of a practice, because survival depended upon the acceptance of a changing medical culture that valued saving money, not people. These kinds of things deeply vexed me. I questioned how I could be different. How could I go through such rigorous training and not only come out alive, but full of passion in my daily encounters as a practicing physician? So, in 1997, with my psychology degree in hand from the University of Colorado, I set out on a quest. I wanted to discover my life's purpose.

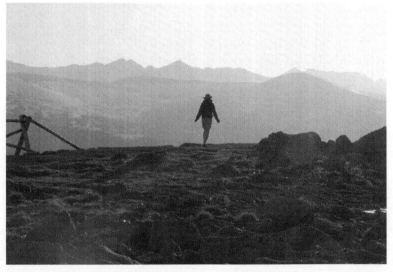

A Journey Into The Unknown

Herpes in the Himalayas

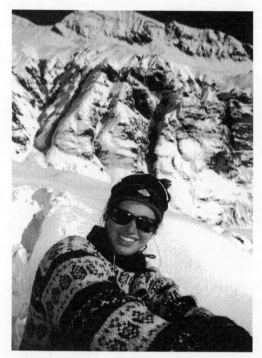

Me at Annapurna Base Camp, Nepal

Working as a sailing instructor, waiting tables, and teaching indoor rock climbing, I saved up enough money throughout college for my dream post-graduation European backpacking adventure. I was driven by a vow to return to Europe after having lived as a high school foreign exchange student with a Portuguese family. As I researched and consumed books about solo woman travelers, my sister anxiously wished that I would find someone to join me. It had not yet occurred to me to invite her; she was living hand-to-mouth as an artist in New York City. I was absolutely shocked when she accepted my invitation to come along. She and I were the best of friends, and I knew that this would be an adventure of a lifetime for both of us. The thought of her baby sister traveling solo across the world was just enough of a nudge for her to commit to a two-month whirlwind tour of Europe.

Michelle and I hit the continent with an insatiable appetite for foreign cultures and traditions. We were explorers at heart, taking in all of the beauty, architecture, art, landscapes, and music that we could reasonably process—and sometimes a bit more. We were the best of traveling companions, often joking that we functioned like an old married couple despite living out of our backpacks. As the trip unfurled, we learned to practically read each other's minds as we rolled in and out of different situations. We developed complementary roles: Michelle navigated us through subways and bus schedules, became my personal docent at art museums and galleries, and kept me laughing with her Carol Burnett–style humor. I pulled the two of us into unplanned adventures and off-the-beaten-path discoveries, somehow getting us by with only a loose command of foreign languages.

We smelled the roses and picnicked under the Eiffel Tower; ate Mozart balls (a scrumptious chocolate delight in Salzburg); explored the largest system of ice caves on the planet in Werfen, Austria; participated in the largest party in the world in Munich, Germany, during Oktoberfest; went spelunking in caves beneath a castle on the Rhine in Germany; soaked in traditional Turkish baths in Hungary; sunbathed nude in Santorini, Greece; and watched the sun set over the Coliseum.

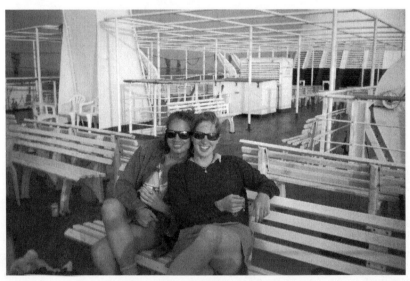

Michelle and Me, Greece

After living out of our backpacks for a month, traveling near and far—Spain, Greece, Italy, France, Germany, Hungary, the Czech Republic, the

Netherlands, Switzerland, and Austria—Michelle got news from New York that she had been hired for a production of *A Chorus Line* in Hawaii. She cut her trip two weeks short and flew back to New York to resume her career in musical theater. Her calling had come calling. I felt that mine was still over the horizon.

Having become very comfortable with traveling light and being on the move, I wanted to stretch my dollars and expand my consciousness. I felt like a true globetrotter as I collected more stamps in my passport, visiting places that had only been images in my mind and wearing the soles of my leather boots thin.

I was beginning to feel like I was the genie in the bottle of my own life. I started to dream the big dream of the mountaineer—to witness the breathtaking beauty of the Himalayan Mountains. One day, while walking across the famous Bosphorus Bridge (a bridge in Istanbul, Turkey, that connects Europe to Asia) for the umpteenth time, I posed a big what-if to myself. What if I could take a flight to Kathmandu? I had always wanted to go to Nepal, but to bring the dream into reality seemed outlandish at the time. Maybe it was the soil of Asia or the call of antiquity that spurred my intrigue. I crossed that bridge several more times before I finally made the decision and booked my flight—a one-way, student-rate ticket from Istanbul to Kathmandu with stops in Bahrain, Saudi Arabia, and Thailand.

The *Lonely Planet Nepal* book I had read before the flight had strongly recommended sitting on the right side of the plane in order to get the best views of the Himalayan Mountains during the approach. I was so excited that I nearly trampled two Indian men while switching sides in the cabin. Louis Armstrong's "What a Wonderful World" was playing on my Walkman as the plane hovered over Mount Everest. I peered down at the snowcapped mountains below, and a tear trickled down my face. Chills ran down my spine. It was magnificent beyond measure.

Kathmandu captured my heart and tickled all of my senses. Everywhere I looked, I saw art in motion. I trusted my head to be the camera and my eyes to be the lens; I felt that there was no way that mechanical photography could capture the essence of this place—a majestic land populated by some of the most gracious, loving people I had met in all of my travels. Even their eyes were soft and inviting. As I peered through the smoke of incense and haze of dirt, it was more like a dream than a reality. The air was dry and smelled of dung and spice. As

I walked the streets, my eyes alit on breathtaking *thangkas*: embroidery and silk paintings delicately accented with twenty-four-karat gold. Some were painted with the beards of monks, who traded their art for food and clothing. Time came to a halt in the spaciousness that I felt while walking the narrow streets and gawking at the art, temples, *sadhus*, and candlelit shrines. I became lightheaded from all of the excitement and energy. At the end of each day, I would close my eyes and thank God for the experience.

While getting my bearings, I began inquiring about trekking in the mountains. Sherpas (local mountain guides) had shops on every corner, engaging travelers to book adventure trips for world-class white-water rafting, jungle tours, and mountain treks. Most tours were significantly cheaper than what their counterparts would charge in the States, but I felt confident that I could trek without the help of a guide.

Trekking was much different than the hiking and backpacking I had done in Utah and Colorado. Each little mountain village in Nepal was connected by hundreds, if not thousands, of single-track walking trails. These trails were an ancient hiking autobahn of sorts for the exchange of goods and services. The locals had built a tourism industry based on small guesthouses and teahouses where travelers could rest their heads, drink some chai, and eat a hot meal at virtually any point along their journey.

I had arrived in Nepal in December. Winter was quickly approaching, and I needed to find a trekking partner, rent a puffy jacket, and apply for a trekking permit before the coming weather put the kibosh on my plans.

My basic plan was inspired by some advice from Tanya, an Australian woman I met while in Turkey. She assured me that I could find a trekking partner on the announcement board at the trekkers' mecca, the Kathmandu Guest House. It was the place to meet up with fellow globetrotters who wanted to explore the surrounding mountains. The Internet hadn't yet overtaken this old-school way of arranging an expedition. You posted an ad on the board and hoped that someone would show up at your proposed time for a meet-and-greet over tea.

After several cups of tea, I met Peter. He had no destination in mind and was easily persuaded by my vision of undertaking one of the most picturesque treks in the world—the sixteen-day Annapurna Base Camp trek. I was lured by its terraced farmland, hot springs, a narrow gorge, and an impressive, glaciered cirque with a panoramic view of ten mountains over

19,500 feet. I can't say that Peter and I had an instant connection, but he was the only one willing to face the challenges of early winter in the Himalayan Mountains with me.

If you pictured Peter as a brawny, steely mountain man when I mentioned him, you are quite far from the truth. A native of Switzerland, Peter was tall and lanky, with a sadness in his eyes and a propensity for the poetry of Tagore. He was a smoker, and I doubt that he had ever done anything athletic before arriving at these mystical mountains. As destiny would have it, I later came to trust Peter as much as the Swiss Army knife in my backpack.

Peter and I immediately applied for our trekking permit, and within twenty-four hours we were on a hair-raising bus ride to Pokhara. Once there, we hit the trail. The clouds hung low in the valley, and the air smelled of earth. Mounds of rice were scattered throughout the terraced fields. All the homes were built from straw and mud; the floors were barren. Dung baked on the rooftops, to be burned later for fuel. I was greeted by ear-to-ear smiles from local children, who carried on their backs baskets twice their size filled with daily staples. Their feet were worn, muddy, and cracked. Quite a contrast to my Gore-Tex leather alpine boots and fancy backpack.

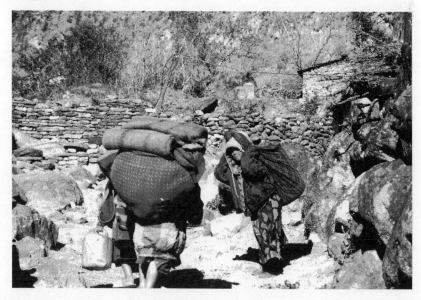

Nepali Children

Trekking up to ten hours a day, I quickly got to know Peter. I resigned myself to his pace, which was much slower than mine, and used the extra time to take in the awe-inspiring beauty that surrounded us at every turn. Some of my fondest memories were moments that passed in complete silence before one of these vistas. The in and out of my breath became my mantra, steadily driving my boots up the mountain path to the summit at Annapurna Sanctuary.

The days were long and sometimes treacherous. We were left exhausted each day by the high-altitude conditions, where each breath became an act of will. Just as soon as we would summit one mountain pass, another would tower in the distance. The terrain was varied: muddy jungles, rice paddies, waterfalls, and exposed rock faces that dropped into a raging, icy river below. Some travelers we met along the way were forced to retreat due to high-altitude sickness. The higher we climbed, the thinner the crowds became. After five days, we finally reached our ultimate destination: the high-altitude Annapurna Base Camp, at 13,500 feet.

Blueberry skies above starkly contrasted the shimmering, white, and jagged 26,000-foot peaks that surrounded us in every direction. It didn't last long. We were hit by a storm. For the next several days, I awoke to the booming of avalanches and the scraping of snow shovels by the workers outside my door. Every day they dug Peter and me out of our room from the several feet of snow that had accumulated the night before. There was no electricity or running water. Even the outhouse had to be dug out several times a day. What a winter wonderland!

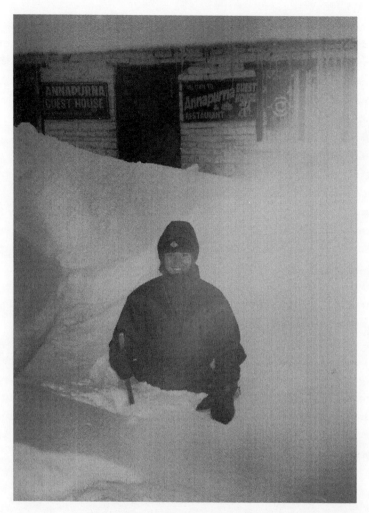

The Snowstorm Of a Lifetime

Days were spent in the guesthouse "living room," which was basically a shack large enough for a picnic table and a few gas camping stoves. The owner of the guesthouse, Didi (which means "grandfather" in Nepalese), spent his days making us *dahl* and rice. Jude (a young trekker from New Zealand), Peter, and I spent hours on end talking, reading, and writing as we huddled around a picnic table. Our feet were warmed by the dicey Nepali method of lighting a camping stove under a picnic table and covering it with a wool blanket. The smell of rotten feet filled the air as my socks began to smolder and smoke.

Feeling the boom in my chest from avalanches and seeing them cascade like waterfalls down the mountains around us made me question whether or not we would make it out alive. A huge storm dumped over eight feet of snow over the course of four days. Our food and fuel resources were dwindling, but the storm did finally cease. The sun came out, and we were able to descend to a safer, lower camp. That's where I met Kevin.

Kevin was a tall, athletic English chap with a Boy Scout–like preparedness for the mountains. Every day, he wore a baseball cap to cover his thinning hair, jeans, and an old, blue, moth-eaten woolen sweater. He smelled of wet, musty wool, like the basement of my childhood. If my memory serves me well, we met in a teahouse on the several-day trek downhill. While Kevin and Peter bantered back and forth with British humor, I found myself focusing on the destination at hand, the Tatapani Hot Springs. I truly did not understand their humor, but the laughter helped me to get my mind off of my painful knee. The stories I had heard about the challenges of the descent being more intense than the uphill battle were ringing true to me. My knees resisted with a click and a throb with each step downhill. I am told that this part of our trek was one of the largest descents in the world—it began atop a soaring mountain and descended to a deep and vast riverbed below. As I limped along on our last day, Kevin offered to carry me. What a romantic gesture, I thought. Although my fairy-tale mind stepped into high gear for a glimpse of fairy dust, I chose to walk it out on my own. Kevin wrapped my knee in his Ace bandage, and I anchored myself in reality as the fairy dust settled.

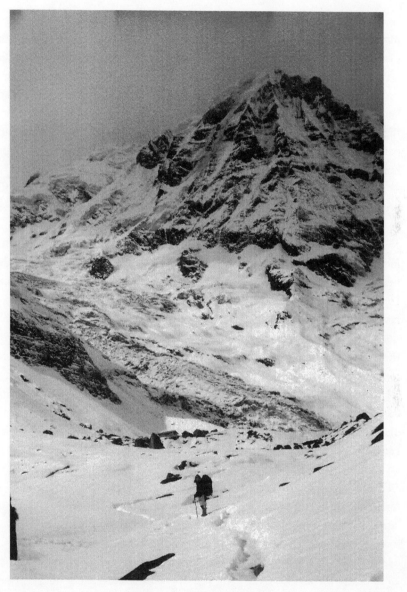

The Long Trek Down

The Tatapani Hot Springs at the lower camp were an oasis of warmth and comfort after having endured the storm's siege on the frigid mountaintops. At that point, I had been away from my family and friends for over four months, and the holidays were approaching. My bones were weary. I found myself longing for a hot shower and a home-cooked meal. I spent hours reminiscing about Christmases past: listening to the Osmonds' Christmas album, dancing with my sister, trimming the tree, wrapping presents, singing carols, and baking cookies with my mother. I missed our family caroling parties, with their jingling bells and silly hats. I would be celebrating my first Christmas away from home. For the first time in my life, I realized that I had been given all the gifts in life that I could ever have dreamed of: a loving family, wonderful friends, a beautiful home, an education, and so much more.

Kevin, Peter, and I spent Christmas Eve day lounging around the hot springs and soaking up sunshine. As day turned to night, my life was forever changed. My heart ached for my family. Unfortunately, paprika chicken and the *tongba* beer (homemade millet beer drunk through slit-metal straws) were no substitute for Mom's cooking during the holiday festivities. After dinner, Kevin and I took a walk back down to the springs. I felt a bit uncomfortable with the way he was looking at me, so I wrapped myself up in a sarong and suggested we look for our friends. That feeling should have been enough of a sign to stay clear.

I could hear some singing in the distance. Tracking the sound, we found a rowdy crowd of Polish men drinking cheap brandy and singing Christmas carols. Kevin began leaning into me as we swayed back and forth, raising our glasses to the cacophonous rendition of "O Christmas Tree" in drunken Polish. One of them was dressed up as St. Nick, bringing the house down with his antics.

Although I had relaxed enough to let Kevin put his arm around me, all I could really think about was a slice of chocolate cake from the local teahouse. So I slipped away, alone in the darkness. The air was cool and laden with sadness. It had sunk in that I was several thousand miles away from home, and for the first time since I had left the US, I was genuinely, deeply homesick. The sound of my flip-flops on the narrow dirt road was all I could hear as I navigated my way through piles of mule dung to seek comfort in that cake.

Within fifteen minutes, Kevin had tracked me down and found me sitting alone with my chocolate cake. We made our way back down to the water, and our playful connection bubbled over into kissing. His hands began to wander all over my body, which was only covered by a bikini and a sarong. His lips began to follow his hands. My heart started to pound.

I felt suddenly that a boundary had been crossed, and told him no. For a brief time, he kissed me south of the border. That was the thirty seconds that changed my life forever. I issued the final no, pushing him away. I just didn't want to share myself with a complete stranger. It felt like a mockery of the true affection I craved. I felt like a sad little girl. I missed my sweet ex-boyfriend back in Colorado. I walked to bed alone.

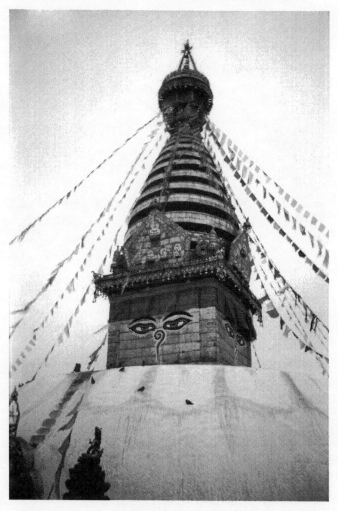

Katmandu, Nepal

My First Herpes Outbreak

Our trip was winding down. It was day twenty-four of our travels and time for Peter and I to make our way back to Kathmandu. Kevin joined us for the next few days of hiking. During that time, a small patch of pin-sized, painful, itchy blisters formed on my genitals. I was totally freaked out. My mind immediately went to the fever blister that Kevin had had on his lips when we were in the high country trekking together. Could it be? Could I have contracted herpes from just a few seconds of oral-genital contact? Maybe it was some "funk" in the hot springs. My mind was racing. Should I tell anyone? It would be a few more days before I could get to a doctor in Kathmandu. I was miserable. The movement of hiking made the symptoms worse. The glands in my neck were swollen, I had a sore throat, and I felt like I had the flu. My muscles ached, and it took every bit of energy I had to hide my crisis from Peter.

Peter's slow, deliberate pace no longer annoyed me. For the first time, we were perfectly paced: the chipper, smiley, optimistic adventurer and the sarcastic, sullen, scholarly pessimist. We found grace in our differences, having spent hundreds of hours sparring intellectually and testing each other's perspectives on life. Hours spent hiking and exploring in mutual reverence of the breathtaking landscape, traversing rigorous terrain and surviving a snowstorm of a lifetime had deepened our friendship. *Should I confide in him?* I thought. Instead, I turned to Kevin first.

I waited until the fear and sadness inside me was ready to burst before I finally opened up to Kevin. My voice quivered and tears rolled down my cheeks as I revealed to him what I had been going through over the past several days. I gathered my strength and tried to focus mainly on describing my symptoms. He seemed genuinely concerned and agreed to help me find answers. Like most men would do, he immediately went into action mode to try and solve the problem. In the meantime, I privately wallowed in misery and uncertainty.

He called the UK seeking medical advice and sought out a backwater pharmacy in Pokhara to see if we could find something to alleviate my symptoms. I vaguely remember leaving the pharmacy with some topical cream in a small tube. The ingredients and instructions were in another language. I had pretty much given up any hope of my symptoms being something other than herpes. Lost in translation, I decided to wait until we got to Kathmandu to seek English speaking health-care professionals and proper medical attention. Later that evening, Kevin took me out to dinner in hopes of getting my mind off of things. No such luck; I was fixated on the inescapable "forever" of herpes.

New Year's Eve was quickly approaching as we made our way back to Kathmandu. The city was buzzing with excitement. Travelers gathered from around the world to celebrate either the beginning or end of their adventures in Nepal. I had gone from the magic of totally surrendering to my life dreams and living them in each and every moment to feeling like no one would ever love me again and that I would never be able to bear children. I truly felt alone, desolate, angry, frustrated, dirty, confused, and depressed. I just had to tell Peter of my sorrows. I was too exhausted from the act of constantly masking the truth to hide it from him for even one more day.

Rolling back into town, we found a little hotel with a peaceful garden courtyard. It was an oasis from the sensory overload of the streets outside. The stillness of the garden called me forth. The sun shone on my face. The floodgate of tears broke. Peter held me as I shook from my sobs, telling him everything. Our purely platonic relationship was a safe haven for me to unravel.

His first reaction was shock. Then he transformed into an angry, protective big brother—this tall, scrawny young man who didn't have a fighting bone in his body was suddenly threatening to take Kevin out. I was floored by this aggressive response. I thought his head would pop off as he vehemently smoked his cigarette, cursing and practically foaming at the mouth. He was truly pissed off that Kevin had passed this infection onto me. I talked him down, and soon he realized that there was truly nothing either one of us could do to right this ship.

The time had come for me to be examined by a doctor. My mind was swirling with questions that no Web site could answer. (In 1998, there weren't a lot of Web sites about herpes.) And in 1998 the Internet was not as well equipped as it is today. It was Visit Nepal 98, and the whole city was shut down for the celebration. Making our way through thousands of people cheering on the parade, Kevin and I found the flashing red-and-green neon cross that marked the medical clinic. I was nervous about going inside, but I had to get my questions answered.

Two different doctors examined me and confirmed my worst fears. Indeed, it was herpes. Hearing it from a white coat made it official. There

I was, in a third-world country, hearing the worst thing that any doctor had ever told me. Dr. Pandy's strong Indian accent made it almost surreal when she answered my number-one burning (no pun intended) question: "Can you really get genital herpes from thirty seconds of kissing down there?" The answer was a resounding yes.

Over the next few days, the tiny, windowless room back at the hotel became my cave of isolation. I locked myself in my bedroom and lay there, trying to process the full range of human emotion, from anger and denial to grief and shame.

I plugged in my earphones and let Sting and Sarah McLachlan lull me in and out of what seemed to be a dream. How could this be? Why me? Couldn't I go back in time to when I was free to just be me without feeling dirty and sexually numb? I felt like herpes was a thief in the night that had robbed me of my right to find love and happiness. Who would ever love me again? I couldn't pretend anymore. I had the Scarlet H.

My mind traveled back to the time I'd spent meditating high in the Himalayas. The snowstorm had forced me to face myself as the chatter of the world fell away. I had questioned life and death, even including a journal entry about how I would want to be cremated if I died. With crystal clarity, the mountaintops had spoken to me. I was to become a doctor. I knew it from the bottom of my heart.

A Holistic Approach: Looking at Health and Herpes from a Whole Perspective

There is more wisdom in your body than in your deepest philosophies.

—FRIEDRICH NIETZSCHE

My time in Nepal and India gave me a whole different perspective that contrasted sharply with my Western traditional upbringing. If I could find stillness in meditation and yoga, I could certainly cultivate healing my herpes and rebalancing my mind. The practice of meditation brought me right back to those frigid mornings in Nepal, slipping out of my warm sleeping bag in the wee hours of the morning, donning my hat and puffy, sea-foam green jacket, and seeking silence before the sun rose.

At that time, I had never read anything about how to meditate, so I just improvised in the spaciousness and solitude of the Himalayan mountain sanctuary. Each morning the mountain gods would whisper to me and guide me through the practice of sitting. The sound of silence was so deafening, you could almost hear the moisture of your exhalation crystallize. My mind would go blank, my legs would become heavy and tingly, and I could feel my cheeks becoming rigid. A frozen smile would arise as the first rays of sun graced my face.

Whenever I did these practices, I could feel energy moving more fluidly in my body and brain. I would then think more clearly and make better choices for my health. It was evident to me that stress was what fueled the fire of imbalance and wrought havoc on my immune system's ability to keep the herpes virus at bay. I did not want to rely on any drug to mask my true imbalances and weaknesses. I wanted to build up my immunity and learn how to better handle stress. Up until that time, I had never needed any drugs, and I was determined to keep it that way.

After my time in Nepal, I attended the University of Vermont and matriculated from their premedical post baccalaureate program. Upon graduation, I moved to Texas and spent a few more years exploring traditional medical careers. My rationale was that if I could do some "rotations" before I applied to medical school, then maybe I could find my specific calling and could *then* commit to a medical school education. I had yet to discover a specialty that truly sparked my interest in its daily practice, and was committed to finding a mentor for inspiration.

As my meditation and yoga practice became more fully ingrained in my life, I began to further explore healing and alternative medicine. I began to question the model and philosophy of our modern health-care system. I was fascinated by the inner workings of healing and what was truly at play. My commitment to becoming a traditional medical doctor was beginning to fade.

While working for an overworked, disillusioned urologist in Austin, my career path was once and for all chosen for me. While cleaning some surgical supplies, a splash of blood entered my eye. Panicked, I reviewed the chart and discovered the patient's history of hepatitis. My heart stopped, and my life flashed before me. The fear of being infected with hepatitis and possibly HIV ran rampant through my mind. I left work early that day and turned to the Internet for answers to solve my most-pressing questions about the likelihood of my being infected with HIV and hepatitis—*and* my life path of becoming a physician.

After surfing the Web, I took a career aptitude test. To my surprise, it not only suggested medicine and teaching, but it also identified chiropractic as an excellent career choice. I had never seen a chiropractor, and my only touchstone with the profession had been listening to my mother urge my father to stop seeing a chiropractor because of her fear of his getting injured. "He'll break your neck!" she would yell at him. It was this test that catapulted me into discovering chiropractic as a viable option for a career in medicine.

Within months, I met a passionate, inspirational chiropractor, quit my job, got a refund for the MCAT, and matriculated into the Parker College of Chiropractic in Dallas, Texas. It was the perfect fit. I finally found the passion and natural approach to medicine that I was looking for. I never looked back.

Chiropractic philosophy made sense to me. Its foundation was based on the belief that the body is governed by an innate, self-healing intelligence found in all living things. This force is responsible for the organization, healing, and maintenance of the body. As a profession, chiropractors remove interference within the nervous system so that the brain and body can have clear signals of communication. Once the interference is removed, the body has an optimal environment in which to heal. This viewpoint merged seamlessly with what I had been learning in my yoga and meditation practices.

From this philosophy I realized that no doctor had ever healed anything! The truth is that the body makes all of the building blocks to heal itself. Yes, doctors have spent years and years doing surgeries and dispensing drugs, but it is the patient that actually does the healing and mending. I'm not saying that intervention doesn't save lives; what I am saying is that you are more powerful than any doctor. You have the ability to heal anything, even herpes! From my perspective, healing herpes translates into discovering a life where symptoms are manageable and the psychological trauma of the diagnosis has dissipated and been transformed into a peaceful state of surrender. Even after fourteen years, I still have an occasional outbreak, and yet it no longer triggers me emotionally and I know just what to do to heal my symptoms. My philosophy on healing continued to develop during my studies and residency in chiropractic school.

Signposts, Not Symptoms

As I stated above, fourteen years after my initial diagnosis, I still get occasional outbreaks. As a result, my viewpoint on healing herpes is not based on the presence or absence of symptoms. I don't use symptoms as my only gauge to determine whether or not I have healed. When symptoms do occur, I look internally to understand what I need to do in order to manage the symptoms. Maybe I'm not making time for myself, eating well, or sleeping enough. Whatever the case is, I can almost always determine the imbalance that contributed to the outbreaks.

Herpes has become a warning signal on my dashboard of health that life has become too stressful or that my physical body has been pushed beyond its limit of adaptation. Long periods of remission allow us to go about our normal lives without having to think about the virus that inhabits our bodies. Does this mean that we are healed? Not necessarily. I think the healthiest people with herpes are the ones that have learned how to better handle their physical and emotional selves. These are the people whom I believe have healed themselves, because they take great care of their physical bodies, and they don't allow an outbreak to trigger a ride on the herpes emotional roller coaster.

For years, my mentor in chiropractic was Dr. Lance Wright, DC. Lance had been an instructor for Network Spinal Analysis until he went his separate way and created his own approach called Flowtrition. Flowtrition is a technique that allows the practitioner to release tension, blocked emotions, and life experiences in the body through a gentle touch. While studying Flowtrition, I spent every waking minute attempting to wrap my mind around what looked like magic. Patients were reporting life-altering experiences as Lance made gentle contacts along their spines. This was unlike any chiropractic I had been introduced to in school. He was the first person I had ever met who truly treated symptoms as signposts that the body was out of balance.

I felt so blessed when Lance tucked me under his wing and mentored me to the point that he was confident in taking a long-awaited vacation to Belize with his wife while I covered his practice and watched his house. A couple times a year he and his wife, Jeanette, would offer healing retreats for his patients. These three-day retreats took place at an amazing wildlife conservatory called Fossil Rim Wildlife Center in Glen Rose, Texas.

Those retreats were so incredibly important for me. For three solid days, we nourished our bodies with raw, organic food, eliminated caffeine and sugar from our diet, turned off our cell phones and computers, and tuned into the inner workings of our bodies and our connection to the natural world. I spent my days journaling, meditating, walking, swimming, drumming, and receiving hands-on group healing sessions, which would sometimes last late into the evening. At day's end, my friends and I would head out into the night. In addition to the light from our flashlights, we were lit up from the inside, piercing the night with a radiance beyond which our eyes could see. On clear evenings, we delighted in sleeping outside on a yurt deck, overlooking the vast Texas outback. There were many nights when I fell asleep to the sound of coyotes calling.

As peaceful and healing as these retreats were, it was not uncommon for me to experience a herpes outbreak within twenty-four hours of my arrival at the retreat. It would begin as a mild tingling and quickly progress into itchy blisters, which would take a week to heal. I would reach ecstatic states of bliss during the group healing sessions. After this happened a handful of times, I started to realize that even states of utter splendor are stressful on the body, in a strange sort of way. This purging of toxins seemed to push the virus right out from hiding and onto the surface of my skin.

Once I was able to reframe my perspective on healing, I could embrace these outbreaks much more easily. "Maybe this will be the last of it all," I would think. For most, the idea of having symptoms worsen as a healing is a bit counterintuitive. I later noticed that during intense healing sessions with spectacular healing modalities, whether it was Qigong, energy work, or chiropractic, my herpes would be triggered. I now respond to these outbreaks as a signpost that either my body is too stressed or that I am healing on a deeper level and that quite possibly the outbreak is my body's attempt to kill off the virus and release it. Strange? Yes, you might think so, but just take a moment to consider the perspective that an increase in symptoms could be related to healing as opposed to regressing. I rarely have these outbreaks anymore, and I believe that this is the result of my cultivating a strong immune system in addition to my healthy, peaceful perspective on living with herpes.

A Healing Crisis: Are Your Symptoms Getting Worse?

A healing crisis occurs when there is an increase in physical and/or emotional symptoms during times of intense healing. In the general view of Western medicine, healing is associated with a decrease in symptoms as opposed to an increase in symptoms. A healing crisis might seem a bit out of the ordinary, because there will always be an increase in symptoms before one gets better. Even with herpes. Let me give you an example to further explain the process.

Your body is an accumulation of life experiences and emotions. Each and every experience you have ever had, on some level, has been stored in your body. An elephant never forgets, so the saying goes; neither does your body. Your body holds on to all of your life experiences, including diseases, illness, trauma and emotional turmoil. This is all well and good when your life is a box of chocolates, but what happens when crisis strikes? During high levels of stress, your body begins to release different hormones than it does when things are going well. As the stress loads increase and the body can no longer handle it, the efficiency of your system as a whole begins to break down. Muscles get tight, immunity decreases, digestion slows, toxins begin to build up, brain function diminishes and your body goes into breakdown mode, much like a car can break down on the side of the road. Each person responds to breakdown mode with different emotions. This breakdown or crisis might lead to high blood pressure, low back pain, diarrhea, headaches, cancer or any number of illnesses. The breakdown could also be a mental breakdown or a bout of depression.

Breakdown mode is like the "straw that broke the camel's back." In these situations, the body can no longer function as normal and the goal of the body is to have you do something different: eat better, sleep more, get more nutrients in your diet, change your body mechanics at work, or decrease the stress in your life. During crisis mode, you can no longer ignore your symptoms and just put tape over the blinking engine light. This down time in crisis is often the perfect opportunity for you to stop, begin listening to your body, and start healing.

Each major crisis in your life is stored like the layers of an onion, where the core is the beginning of your life and the outer layers are your most recent years. A good healer will begin working with the outermost, most recent layer of your life. This is often why you sought care in the first place.

If your symptom is something that has been chronic, it is most probably linked to an imbalance from times past. During intense holistic healing, the body begins to re-pattern itself, so that new neural connections are made and balance is restored. These healing crisis symptoms are revealed in a reverse chronological order, much like pulling back the layers of an onion.

Let's say that five years ago you had a bout of cancer, and fifteen years ago you broke your arm. In this case, you might re-experience the symptoms of cancer as your body completes that layer of healing. During this new layer of integration and healing, your body will begin to release toxins and emotions associated with the original trauma. In this case, maybe a rash might form as the body releases stored toxins from chemotherapy. The next major healing crisis in your journey might appear as an increase in pain in your arm. Maybe your arm never fully repaired itself and now the body wants to address this injury because it has the available nutrients and energy. As your body builds new material pathways and breaks down scar tissue, you are left with an arm that is better than ever.

The good news is that these healing crisis symptoms generally only last for a few days, or up to a week. It is not uncommon for emotions to also be released as the body reintegrates and heals. Unfortunately, there are no guidelines I have for you to distinguish a healing crisis from a new injury or a remedy that might not be working for you. Spend time in reflection and listen to your intuition as a guiding force.

If you are just beginning to heal your herpes, be sure to give a remedy some time to work, and don't be surprised if your symptoms get worse before they get better. It is quite possible that the remedy or exercise might be causing the virus to be killed off in large numbers. This could lead to an increase in symptoms as your body attempts to push the virus out of your body from a dormant state to an active state. This *could* be a healing response. Healing naturally works from the inside out and sometimes requires more patience. You always have the option of changing your regimen.

The Impact of Our Emotions on Symptoms

When I met my husband, Richard, I had reached a point in my healing where I was only occasionally having herpes outbreaks on my face. My main triggers had been pared down to pure bliss and dating. This probably sounds totally ridiculous. Peruse any online forum or book about herpes, and I challenge you to find these as triggers. As luck would have it, and not surprisingly so, I am one of a unique breed of carriers—or at least I thought so until I spoke with several more women with herpes who had similar experiences.

Dating Richard initially increased my outbreaks to the point where I was getting a sore on my face at least twice a month. They followed no pattern with my menses, the food I ate, or any other common triggers. It seemed that whenever I was interested in dating someone, the outbreaks would reoccur. It's as if the love hormones would begin to trickle throughout my body and elicit an outbreak. If I liked someone, it would be like the same feeling I got when I was a little girl and I had a crush on a boy. Sometimes, before I even had a chance for a second date, the sore would rear its ugly head. When it did, I would have to explain what that thing was on my face. I did not feel comfortable having "the Talk" at such an early stage in a relationship. It felt like it was the only thing I saw when I looked in the mirror. I will never forget the day Richard asked if I could put some makeup on it before we went out to a social gathering. I was mortified, and apparently he was embarrassed, too, because he knew what it was.

When I talked to other women, they also said that even the thought of dating would elicit the onset of symptoms. I can remember being so fearful of another genital outbreak after going on a date that I would start to feel tingling down there and would get out a small mirror to see if there were any sores. I would constantly question whether or not the tingling was in my head. At times I thought I was going crazy. I would check, check, and recheck to see what was going on down there, and of course I would wash my hands several times a day. I was conscious enough to know that if things went well, I would have to have "the Talk," and this fear was driving the show. Try *not* to think of a pink elephant, and sure enough, a pink elephant appears.

Is There a Magic Bullet for Herpes?

As a practicing chiropractor, I always made certain that I treated the whole person and not just the symptoms. Two people could show up with the exact same symptoms, and yet they would respond differently to each healing modality. Herpes is no different. There was a time when my quest for a cure muddied my mind and caused me to question whether or not there *might* be a magic bullet for herpes. For years, I scoured the Internet, attempting to discover the cure, only to find my pocketbook dwindling and my hopes diminishing. I must have spent thousands of dollars with acupuncturists, Ayurvedic practitioners, Qigong masters, pills, salves, psychics, Reiki masters, chiropractors, tonics, and Web site scams, hoping to cure the incurable.

At some point, I surrendered to the truth that herpes was with me for life. I quit spending money chasing the next new healing method. I knew that healing was an inside job and that there were no magic pills. During my process of "sweet surrender", in the fall of 2008, I had a hair analysis done with a thirty-year expert in the field, Dr. Lawrence Wilson, MD. I turned to him for guidance for detoxification of heavy metals and mineral balancing, but not for my herpes, per se. He designed a vitamin and mineral program for me based on my results and made several other recommendations. He became my nutritional mentor, and it was under his tutelage that I began offering the same services to my patients.

After I had been on the program for several months, I realized that my outbreaks had ceased. I went from having a few outbreaks a month to nearly none at all. It took me a long while to realize what had changed. I was hoping that my patients with herpes would have the same results I did, only to find that they didn't. Some would improve while others did not. "Why?" I asked myself. It was because a nutritional program only addressed one leg of the Triad of Health, which, in its entirety, includes a physical (diet, nutrition, and structure), a mental (thoughts), and an emotional/spiritual component. When any element of this triad is weak, it affects the whole. For me, the weak links of the Triad were in the physical and the emotional components. The reality was that Dr. Wilson's program did not have any magic, either. So, why did I get such great results?

I believe that there were a few things in the program that, combined with my readiness to heal, made all of the difference for me. The program helped me to detoxify my body and to replenish it with some key vitamins and minerals. In addition, a huge contributor to my healing—or, shall I say, managing—my herpes was that I had found a place of surrender and self-love. This speaks to the emotional component of the triad. I believe to this day that *this* was truly the magic in my journey of self-discovery. Just like I was ready to love my husband Richard, I had also found a safe place to love myself. Believe me, there were times when outbreaks on my face, the size of a quarter, made me question my self-love.

It was through herpes that I was able to develop a stronger compassion for those less fortunate, especially with physical and emotional illnesses. I developed more self-worth within partnership, with myself and with others. Once I was able to totally love myself and to surrender to the outbreaks, herpes went into hiding. Self-love was the elixir for me, and if I could bottle that, I would be a billionaire many times over. Once we can find love and compassion for ourselves, we are then, and only then, able to discover it in others and to share our love with the world.

Eastern and Western Perspectives on "Healing" Herpes

Western medicine = modern medicine
Eastern medicine = traditional, holistic, and alternative medicine

Eastern medicine is rooted in a holistic or whole body approach. The physical, emotional, and spiritual states of an individual are all equally important in evaluating, managing, and treating an individual. Imagine a hologram where every individual part represents the whole. It is impossible to break down a hologram into individual parts. Let's say you have a hologram of an apple. If you cut the apple hologram in half, you are not left with two halves; you are left with two whole apples. You can demolish a hologram, but even a minute piece of the original will still reflect the whole!

Holistic medicine and its premises are no different than a hologram. You can't heal a person by just examining and treating one part of their body, because everything is so interconnected. For example, you might be able to "fix" a person's heart by treating a blockage with surgery. This is more of a Western approach, which focuses only on the physical symptom at hand, the blockage. This modern approach to medicine views the body as individual parts that need to be fixed. The weakness in this approach is that unless the underlying cause is addressed, the symptom will arise again in a similar or different form.

In Western medicine, an individual might have a half a dozen doctors who specialize in one specific thing, making it incredibly difficult to locate a disease and find a lasting solution. It's as if our "parts" don't communicate with one another, and a section is quarantined. Within the eyes of many Western doctors, the sum of our parts equals the whole.

In Eastern medicine, health comes from an innate return to balance in the system. "Fixing" a problem entails a deep investigation of the environment that led to the imbalance or physical symptom and then going deeper to where the root of the problem lies. What were the person's daily habits? How did their other organs function? Did they eat well? Were they stressed at work? Did they exercise? What were their families' health backgrounds? What was going on in their personal lives? These are just a handful of the many questions that need to be answered in order to understand the emotional, spiritual, and physical ailments of an individual person.

From a holistic perspective, herpes cannot be healed by a medicine that solely focuses on killing the virus. You must consider all the conditions that were present when you contracted the virus: your mental and physical states, as well as your emotional and spiritual health. Your medicine will be revealed once you discover the weaknesses within your whole being. What part of your Triad of Health is weak? Is it the physical body, mental body, or spiritual/emotional body? The main premise of Western medicine is that healing comes from the outside in, as opposed to the inside out. In the outside-in approach, one believes that health is derived from external means: doctors, surgeries, and drugs. In turn, a lack of respect develops for the power of the body in its ability to heal itself. As patients, we find ourselves victims of the life we have been dealt and the genes that we carry instead of actively involving ourselves in the healing process.

If you are at the beginning of your journey with herpes, you probably relate to herpes as the villain that lives in your body and needs to be eradicated. A Western thought would be "Kill the virus," whereas an Eastern thought might be "What is out of balance here and how can we reclaim wholeness?" I invite you to step back and surrender to your current reality. You can choose to spend the rest of your life looking for your health "out there," or you can powerfully choose to find your health from "in here." This is how I choose to take responsibility for my health and to live, love, and thrive! It is your choice, and if you choose to look "out there," you might be able to mask your symptoms. But if you look inside yourself, you will gain strength, rebuild your immunity, and find a power greater than any drug. This is why I believe herpes can be your teacher.

If you do choose to use drugs to manage your herpes, I believe a fundamental understanding of how they work is important. Western medicine's approach to herpes is to use drugs that disrupt the virus's ability to replicate, decreasing the frequency and severity of outbreaks and speeding up healing times. This is done at the genetic level. Just a few weeks ago I spoke with an STD specialist who worked at an STD clinic in Denver. He said, on average, antiviral medications were able to speed healing time in his herpes patients by a day. Indeed, his practice was reflective of the norm, and to me, this "speedy recovery" of one less day did not seem to be that impressive. There have also been some prescriptions that have been shown to decrease viral shedding.[1] These products are taken both internally and topically on the skin. Occasionally, I will come across someone whom I believe, short term, can benefit from antiviral drugs until we can balance out his or her body naturally. As with any drug, there are risks involved. Specifically, Valtrex (an antiviral) is considered safe, but so is aspirin, and death is a potential risk with even aspirin.

The risk of any drug is often greater than the risk of a natural plant or alternative medicine. Your body recognizes a natural substance better than something made in a lab. I personally do not feel comfortable taking a pill that disrupts the herpes virus at the level of DNA, our genetic makeup. If a holistic practitioner hands you a "natural" pill, a garlic clove, or a mushroom capsule, it is much better than a chemically based drug. However, this is still an external approach and comes from the perspective that one remedy works for all individuals. A truly holistic practitioner will consider your unique experience when recommending solutions for herpes, as this book does.

Let's take a look at herpes drugs and how they are portrayed in our media. I remember the first time I saw a commercial for the prescription drug, Valtrex. A happy couple skipped through a field of flowers, making the audience believe that this was what it was like to have herpes. It's as

---

1 Viral shedding occurs when the herpes virus is active and replicating at the surface of the skin. During this time, the virus can be transmitted, even though other noticeable symptoms might not be present.

if these drug companies are saying, "If you take this drug, you are bound to live happily ever after." I hate to be the bearer of bad news, but you are responsible for your own health, and once you realize it's an inside job, you will be much better off. Hiding the symptoms and never dealing with the emotions that come along with the virus will only leave you a time bomb waiting to explode at the drop of a hat. While viewing another commercial for Valtrex, I realized that 75 percent of the time was spent verbally disclosing the side affects. If you do your research, you will discover that the most common drugs to treat herpes have a litany of side affects and warnings. Valtrex, for example, warns patients:

Kidney failure and nervous system problems are not common, but can be serious in some patients taking VALTREX. Nervous system problems include aggressive behavior, unsteady movement, shaky movements, confusion, speech problems, hallucinations (seeing or hearing things that are really not there), seizures, and coma. Kidney failure and nervous system problems have happened in patients who already have kidney disease and in elderly patients whose kidneys do not work well due to age. **Always tell your healthcare provider if you have kidney problems before taking VALTREX. Call your doctor right away if you get a nervous system problem while you are taking VALTREX.**

Common side effects of VALTREX in adults include headache, nausea, stomach pain, vomiting, and dizziness. Side effects in HIV-1-infected adults include headache, tiredness, and rash. These side effects usually are mild and do not cause patients to stop taking VALTREX.

Other less-common side effects in adults include painful periods in women, joint pain, depression, low blood cell counts, and changes in tests that measure how well the liver and kidneys work.[2]

Wow! We have become so accustomed to hearing about the risks of using drugs that we tune them out and disconnect from their warnings. To see the risks in print can be shocking. I have read the ingredients of some of the "cure" products found online and have also been shocked by what I

---

2 Patient Information Leaflet for Valtrex.

discovered. One such claim made by a product called MMS2, or Miracle Mineral, had 28 percent sodium chlorite, which is the equivalent of *industrial-strength bleach*. Of course this would kill off some of the herpes virus—along with everything else in its path! Other topical ingredients have been known to burn the skin. So, if there is any copy that mentions cure, beware!

Herpes "Cures": Is the FDA Really Protecting Us?

The FDA is finally cracking down on Internet companies that are making false claims about herpes. In May of 2011, the FDA issued warnings to companies making "false" or misleading claims that holistic drugs such as Medavir, Herpaflor, and Viruxo "cure" herpes.[3] However, after reviewing some of the companies that are currently under the scrutiny of the FDA, I have discovered that some of the products are composed of legitimate therapeutic ingredients. As a doctor, healer, and herpes patient, I wonder if these companies will be shut down because they are getting such great results with their products. Such results would pose as direct competition for the pharmaceutical companies.

This FDA crackdown on these companies leaves me both thrilled and a bit fearful. I am thrilled because it has been a long time coming for companies using the word "cure" to be required to stand behind their claims. If there is a natural cure out there, I want to know about it. I do hope that we can continue to reap the benefits of easy access to quality natural products. With that said, selling snake oil as a "cure for herpes" should be illegal.

The reason I am also fearful is that I don't trust the FDA to protect us from any harm. There are several things in our marketplace that have been proven time and again to be detrimental to our health, and yet the FDA turns a blind eye. The United States is light years behind Europe when it comes to protecting its citizens from truly toxic substances. Most of Europe (97 percent) does not fluoridate their water, nor do they tolerate toxic food additives like GMOs (genetically modified organisms) or pesticides. The use of fluoride in our water is a great example of how the FDA does not always protect us and will, in fact, allow the interests of big business and profits to outweigh its commitment to our health.

3 Mathew Perrone, "Feds Take Action against Bogus Herpes Cures," Associated Press (ABC News), Washington, May 3, 2011.

Very few Americans know that the safety of fluoride was never researched before approval. Fluoride toxicity has been linked to several adverse affects on the human body, including brain damage, osteoarthritis, bone weakening, lower IQs, birth defects, enzyme inhibitions, and more.[4] Why would our government place this toxic substance in our water? The answer is quite clear: to find a dumping ground and use for a byproduct of many industrial processes. Although the toxicity of fluoride is debated in the United States, the European government deemed its safety questionable enough to remove it from their water system.[5]

I use these as examples for those who have never questioned the protection of our FDA. The real question is this: why is the FDA getting involved with herpes supplements now? What are their intentions? Are they truly attempting to protect the American people, or are they financially being compensated and wooed by drug companies who would much rather have our dollars spent on drugs and vaccines?

Every now and then, I receive a barrage of e-mails explaining potential threats of Americans losing our rights to purchase and use over-the-counter natural remedies. Since 1962, the Codex Alimentarius Trade Commission has been hard at work trying to limit access to unadulterated food and high-potency nutrients. This United Nations group was formed by WHO (the World Health Organization) and FAO (the Food and Agricultural Organization) to create international standards or "food rules" to protect the safety of its consumers. Under the Codex Alimentarius (Latin for "food rules"), vitamin C, an inexpensive natural remedy that is used as an immune builder, antioxidant, and anti-inflammatory, has been reclassified from a nutrient to a toxin at levels above the RDA (recommended daily allowance) at 75 mg/day for females and 90 mg/day for men.

Under the Codex Alimentarius, anything sold above the RDA dosage would require a doctor's prescription. This would be much more expensive for consumers and would make preventive health a luxury only available to the wealthy. To put this into perspective, a therapeutic dose of vitamin C is frequently used at levels one hundred times the RDA, if not more without toxic side effects. In places like Canada and Europe, Codex Alimentarius laws are in place. My concern here is that eventually doctors will hold all of our rights to the pursuit of optimal health, and that

---

4 Found online at http://www.holisticmed.com/fluorides.

5 Found online at http://www.fluoridealert.org/fluoride-facts.

pharmaceutical companies will hold the purse strings to all of our natural alternatives to prescription drugs. I think the FDA involvement brings to light a very important question I must ask. Who is responsible for your health anyway? Is it the government? Will they protect you?

Are you waiting for alternative healing practices to be proven? Research takes tons and tons of money, and given enough money and politics, any data can be manipulated to create a favorable outcome. I am not against science, but there are healing practices that science might never "prove"—and yet they are still valid and therapeutic. It is the behemoth pharmaceutical industry backing prescription drugs versus the healers and individual practitioners supporting alternative medicine. If you wait for a natural remedy to be "proven," you will stay behind the eight ball and remain sick. If you don't realize this, it is about time you do.

It is critical for you to begin to question your viewpoints on health, healing, and our current health-care system. The old ways of looking at your health might not serve you in your healing journey. Allow herpes to be your wake-up call—your opportunity to become more educated about what optimal health might look like for you. Chances are, you will stop following the pack and start thinking for yourself. You will keep your best interest in mind when it comes to your health. You can become the most educated about your particular ailments and imbalances. Remember, doctor means teacher, and as your teacher, I will allow you to take the lead.

Consciously Implementing Change: Lianna's Story

One afternoon, while Lianna —a dear friend of mine—and I were hiking, I shared my personal experience with herpes. I told her that although I had learned and implemented everything there was to know about the physical management of my symptoms, I still got outbreaks. It took me a long time to realize that negative thought patterns and self-limiting beliefs would almost always trump an impeccable diet and supplement regimen. It shocked me to realize how powerful my thoughts were, and how they could hinder my healing progress. Herpes loves thoughts of rejection, shame, isolation, and victimhood. While this discovery is extremely frustrating for someone who suffers from herpes, on the flip side, it is also uplifting to know how much power there is in positive thoughts.

As our conversation evolved, Lianna let her guard down and began to share a very personal story with me. Several years before she met her husband, she was diagnosed with genital herpes. While reading the paper one day, she discovered an advertisement for a drug company that was seeking volunteers with genital herpes. She jumped at the chance to participate in a study that had the potential to "cure" her outbreaks. Hope was on the horizon, finally. If she could just get her symptoms under control, maybe she could find love. She was eager to find her life partner and decided that this trial would give her the opportunity to heal her herpes before she met her soul mate.

Shortly after reading the ad, Lianna contacted the research team and committed to participating in round one of the trials to be held in Las Vegas. With her spirits high, Lianna booked a round-trip ticket from Colorado, reserved a hotel room, and secured time off from work. For the first time ever, she flawlessly followed the dietary recommendations provided by her doctor. No nuts, alcohol, coffee, sugar, chocolate, or caffeine. It was a very trying time for her because coffee and chocolate were two of her greatest joys in life.

As her departure date for Las Vegas neared, Lianna could not stop thinking about her herpes. She had reached a point in healing where she could manage her outbreaks to some degree, but she wanted to be cured for good. Lianna built up a lot of expectations for this new drug to be her saving grace. A week before she left, her plan to go on "vacation" to heal her herpes leaked throughout her work environment, and things began to fall apart. Before she knew it, coworkers were afraid of using the bathroom for fear of sharing the same toilet with her. (Herpes cannot be transmitted on toilet seats.) She was humiliated and devastated!

As she packed her bags, she broke down crying and wondered if she would ever be able to get her herpes under control. She had an outbreak on the day she arrived and was released from the study, which required all participants to be symptom-free. She realized in that moment that her mind was as powerful, if not more powerful, than any recommendations that a doctor could ever make. It was her incessant worry and anxiety surrounding herpes that caused her to go into outbreak mode. She finally understood that it had been months since she had had an outbreak, and it was her thought patterns that had triggered her outbreak.

Lianna had learned a very beautiful lesson. She realized that she had all the tools she needed to manage her outbreaks. She had followed the recommendations from her doctor to a T. The only thing that had changed was her negative thought patterns—something that she could control. She already knew the basics of a healthy diet that could keep her herpes outbreaks at bay and had taken steps to reduce stress and anxiety. Most importantly, she realized that she wasn't interested in a healing method that encompassed modern medicine. She wanted a truly alternative and holistic approach to managing her herpes.

This story exemplifies so many lessons. No matter how well you follow the guidelines for the management of symptoms, never underestimate the power of your thoughts. Positive thoughts and affirmations can help to re-pattern any negative thoughts that might arise from a herpes diagnosis. Herpes allows you the opportunity to be more positive and compassionate toward yourself. Take this time to evaluate your daily thoughts, and see if they lean more toward negativity or positivity. We will talk more about this in chapter four, but for now, it's best to keep a journal to see where you are.

This story also speaks to a holistic viewpoint of herpes versus a modern medical approach. Modern medicine will dispense a pill for your herpes ailment, but it will not address any other imbalances that might be occurring in your body. Holistic medicine looks at you as a whole person with physical, mental, emotional, and spiritual needs. It does not view herpes as the only imbalance in your body. Are your symptoms worse because of a depressed immune system or because of your defeatist mental thought processes? Not every person with herpes is the same, and therefore the remedy for symptom suppression is not the same.

The answers to managing your symptoms might be a combination of things, including dietary changes, supplements, detoxification strategies, stress management, and emotional rebalancing. You might best respond to a daily regimen of meditation, or you might best respond to a strict herpes diet. If you take the time to commit to healing, you will discover what best works for your body.

In her quest for answers, Lianna discovered that she had all of the tools she needed to heal and that her thoughts were the most powerful determining factor of her outbreaks. Take Lianna's story to heart and know that you, too, are more powerful than you give yourself credit for. Be open to the answers that lie within and receptive to herpes-management strategies that take the whole you into consideration.

THREE

The Role of Grief and the Power of Forgiveness in Managing Your Herpes

We must embrace pain and burn it as fuel for our journey.

—KENJI MIYAZAWA

Being diagnosed with herpes has a similar grief cycle to losing a loved one or being diagnosed with a terminal disease. We feel as if we have lost one of the most sacred aspects of our being—our sexual self. Our private, secret garden now seems tainted and damaged. A part of you dies because you can never return to your innocence. You now must carry a social consciousness in regards to your sexual behavior and the potential transmission of the virus.

If you choose to remain in denial, you will probably be plagued by a tremendous amount of suffering. Becoming celibate and rejecting yourself as a sexual being is an option too, but not a healthy one. Even if you had a positive relationship with your sexual self prior to being diagnosed with herpes, it is very challenging to maintain your sexual self-confidence and sexual prowess upon your initial diagnosis. Over time, it is possible to reverse this.

We all desire to be loved, and anything that is perceived as disruptive to our "lovability factor" can directly impact every aspect of our lives—if we allow it to. The grief cycle and emotional healing associated with herpes is a process that occurs over a period of time. For some it might be six months. For others, like myself, it takes years. Each outbreak is an opportunity to look inward and to experience another layer of introspective healing. There is no end to this journey, only several new beginnings.

Flowing with Grief: Integrating Your Emotions

*Magic happens when we are able to stand in
the perfection of our imperfections.*

Healing herpes follows a flow very similar to a river coursing through varied terrain. Sometimes it feels like a Class V river rapid filled with crashing waves, turbulent swells, and daredevil chutes. Other times it slows nearly to the point of complete stillness, imperceptibly moving like the Mississippi River to Roger and Hammerstein's lyrical song, "Ol' Man River." Sometimes it feels like your whole world is turning upside down and you feel chaos in your body. Other times you will feel brackish, depressed, and numb. All of these emotional states are totally normal.

Experiencing these diabolically different emotions can be challenging, to say the least. After years of investigating these emotional states, I have come to identify six main stages. No two people will go through these stages in the same way, and it is quite common to revisit previous states from time to time. The most important thing to do during these unique stages is to embrace your feelings and be with them.

Moving through grief will embody both ebbing and flowing qualities, as life moves through each tidal change. There is a time to turn inward and to be still and a time to explore movement and externalized emotions.

I have identified these unique stages as Still Periods and Flow Periods. Through stages one, three, and five (explained below), you might naturally feel more shut down or at a standstill. This is the time to follow the guidelines outlined below. Perception of time during these periods of stillness might be warped, akin to the slow, methodical movements of a tortoise. During these times of inward processing, review the recommendations below so that you can best integrate your emotions during these stages of healing.

During a Still Period

Be gentle with yourself.	Watch inspiring movies.
Explore solitude.	Hang with girlfriends.
Take a bath.	Drink herbal tea.
Eat soul food.	Meditate.
Get a massage.	Light candles.
Practice gentle yoga.	Explore art.
Dive deep into a novel.	Reflect and journal.
Get near or in water.	Spend time with animals.
Sit and reflect in nature.	Take up stargazing.

In contrast, the even-numbered stages two, four, and six are filled with energy rising and eager to move and flow. These times can be very productive if you allow the body to outwardly express itself. Support your grieving process by acknowledging and embracing where you are. Don't fight it. During these times of flow, let your hair down and get moving!

During a Flow Period

Exercise.	Punch a pillow.
Communicate your emotions.	Go for a run, hike, or swim.
Lift weights.	Jump!
Sing at the top of your lungs!	Dance.
Listen to music that makes you MOVE!	Take up karate.
Spin around and around.	Go to a boxing class.
Climb a mountain.	Yell underwater.

Now that we have covered the basic energies of the ebb and flow of healing, let us more deeply explore the six major stages of grief.

Stage One: Trauma and Denial (STILL PERIOD)

When you are first diagnosed with herpes, your first reaction is one of shock and denial. You think, "This can't be happening to *me*," and yet it is. You are confused, fearful, restless, stunned, and irrational. You are in a constant state of placing blame, whether it is on yourself or another. It is not uncommon to experience a whole array of emotions, including self-blame, anger, shame, embarrassment, depression, and lack of self-love. You feel disgusting in your own body, which was once a sacred haven for you.

Suffering and the feeling of being separated from the core of your being are central to the first stage of healing. At this point, you are acutely aware that there is something wrong! You might have feelings of "Why me, why now?" I sure did! I was confused and had no connection to my emotions. I felt like a foreigner in my own body!

During Stage One, it is so easy to blame yourself or the person who gave you herpes. You feel you have become a victim to your condition. Each woman has her own story to tell. Maybe your partner knew he or she had herpes and never told you. Maybe you went home after a drunken escapade only to find yourself in bed with a stranger. Or maybe you were falling in love for the first time and you contracted it during your first sexual experience. Whatever the case, you have done no wrong! Herpes knows not who you are or what you do. You are an innocent host, but not a victim.

Stage Two: Feelings of Rage (FLOW PERIOD)

In Stage Two you are pissed off at yourself and the person who gave you herpes. There is no turning back now, and you know it. You realize that you must carry the burden of a sexually transmitted disease, and your life will never be the same. You are ashamed, edgy, and irritable. You might even be taking your anger out on other friends or family members. This is also known as projection. It feels like road rage on your inner highway, and if you don't do something, you will explode. You must embrace this anger and allow it to move through your body. If you stuff it, it will slowly fester, bubble up inside, and eventually explode or further degrade your health.

As women, many of us have never been taught how to express our anger in a healthy way. Our society views women who openly express their anger as bitches, but listen to me: this is a time to call upon your inner bitch and release the anger. But here is the caveat: you must release it through vocalization and movement in a new, healthy way.

Stage Three: Profound and Prolonged Sadness (STILL PERIOD)

Welcome to Stage Three. You now feel as if you have been run over by a steamroller. Your life has come to a complete stop. You feel profoundly sad and numb. Your heart and body feel like they weigh one thousand pounds. Your shoulders are slumped, your feet drag on the floor, and it is hard to make it through each day. All you want to do is sit on the couch with your new best friends, Ben and Jerry, stuffing yourself. Chances are, now is not the time to explore any new flavors; you seek comfort in familiarity. You feel helpless. While the shock has worn off, you don't know where to turn. You don't feel like taking on new activities and hanging with friends; thus, work might be your only social stimulation. If this goes on for more than a few weeks, I highly suggest joining our online herpes community, seeking counseling, or joining a local herpes support group. Have faith; you will get through this, and know that there is light at the end of the tunnel. Be very gentle with yourself, eat well, and make a daily meditation practice a top priority.

Stage Four: Communicating and Reaching Out (FLOW PERIOD)

This is the stage where your energy moves you to make a change. You have spent enough time with your thoughts, and it is time to begin to share your story and gather information, seeking out the resources that you so desperately need. Community is at the core of this stage because through other peoples' stories and statistics, you realize that you truly are not alone in your suffering. You begin to establish meaning in your life and are more armed with power to look inward for answers. You now have an inner dialogue that is more positive than the previous stages.

This is where the turnaround from breakdown to breakthrough can occur. No one desires to feel helpless and all alone. Coming into your community can be extremely healing. Your friends and family can serve as reminders of your true, brilliant nature. Share your story with a loved one who has supported you in times past and knows how to support you in a positive manor. You can begin to rebuild your self-esteem and remember your higher calling and meaning in life. It is cathartic to begin connecting and sharing with others. This will help you to process and integrate your emotions more easily. No longer will you feel so alone on this journey.

While Stage Four is presented as a later part of the journey, this is not always the case. For some, it overlaps with Stage One. Each journey is unique, and if you are more extraverted or verbal, beginning to process Stage Four earlier in your journey is totally appropriate.

Stage Five: Surrender and Acceptance (STILL PERIOD)

This is the stage where you are able to accept and embrace your future. You become more compassionate toward yourself and the person who gave you herpes. Peace begins to replace anger and fear. Forgiving yourself and others becomes a constant practice in this stage. Grief is now lifting, and your life is beginning to return to normal. Your herpes no longer victimizes you.

This is a great time to implement the forgiveness exercise outlined in this book. Spend time surrendering. Let your guard down and learn how to love yourself completely, just as you are, today.

Stage Six: Empowerment (FLOW PERIOD)

Yeah! You are finally able to embrace all of your gifts and envision a life of happiness and sweet surrender. Your willingness to truly live has returned. Now you know the facts about herpes, how it is spread, and what you can do to decrease your outbreaks. You feel empowered and have more control of your life, as you have created your own treatment plan for managing your outbreaks. Emotionally, you feel you are on more stable ground and have a new level of commitment to your health and well-being.

Get It OUT of Your System: Share Your Story!

Over the years I have found that sharing my story has given me the power to find peace in living with herpes. When I step into my power and share my story, it gives other women the opportunity to do the same. I have discovered a huge gap in the state of healing in women who have shared their story as compared to women who have kept it a secret. Women who share are much more able to cope with the "forever" of herpes. There is a tremendous amount of support available to you when you share your story and release your emotions around it. If you keep herpes a secret, then it can become a skeleton in your closet that eats away at your soul, year after year.

I am certain that you will eventually need to share your story with a partner, but do not dismiss the healing power of your sisters—the women in your life who love you and support you. Early on, I told my mother, sister, and best friend about my herpes. They were able to hold me in their hearts and offer me a great deal of strength and compassion.

When we reveal our innermost secrets, especially to other women, a gateway of sorts begins to emerge. This gateway opens up our hearts and allows us to connect to others in a much deeper way. Maybe your best friend or mother has herpes, too, and you would never know it unless you shared your story. Chances are, the woman or women you confide in will feel more connected to you because you entrusted your story to them. When you trust more in them, they will trust more in you. Your inner strength will serve as a mirror for them to find their strength. I can offer a way for you do this right now—consider sharing your story with our community at www.talkaboutherpes.com. In sharing, you will inspire other women to tell their story.

The Act of Forgiveness

Forgive: if you never know forgiveness,
You'll never know the blessings that God gives.

—RUMI

I have spent a lifetime in the world of personal growth and spirituality, and have found the act of forgiveness to be one of the most powerful human acts on the planet. Forgiveness is at the core of many spiritual practices and texts, including one of my favorite books, *A Course in Miracles*. When I think about what it means to forgive, I am reminded of one of my favorite country songs. It talks about burying the hatchet but leaving the handle sticking out. Whenever we get into a fight, we start digging up things that should be long forgotten.

While many can say they practice forgiveness, I have found they've done just that. In other words, people will say that they've forgiven the person who gave them herpes, but more often then not, they superficially try to move on and forget that which they seek to heal—until the next trigger arises or the next potential partner comes around.

This is not forgiveness. To forgive someone means to find total peace within yourself and to remove the charge from the person who needs forgiveness. To forgive is truly to bury the hatchet and walk away, never looking back. In doing so, you will access a power to heal and find a peace that is more powerful than any drug.

Forgiveness Is the Gift You Give Yourself

There can be several layers to forgiveness. While I was still having herpes outbreaks on a consistent basis, I would practice forgiveness as a healing process in and of itself. I intuitively knew that each outbreak was an opportunity for me to practice forgiveness, not just for the person who gave me herpes but for anyone in my life toward whom I was still holding judgment. Once you get into the groove of forgiveness, you might find a whole list of people you need to forgive. Why not hold a whole forgiveness and healing weekend in the privacy of your own home. Light some candles and go for it!

When you forgive, you allow yourself to move on, attaining more freedom in your life. Forgiveness allows you to heal and grow. The simple act of forgiveness can change the course of your whole life. Spiritual and physical laws are at play here. You see, when you change yourself, you change the way others interact with you. And you also impact the life of the person you are forgiving. It's almost like changing the locks on your house. The old key won't work anymore, so people can no longer interact with you in the exact same way. Your buttons and triggers are all reprogrammed. It is a universal law that one small change cannot occur in isolation. You might not notice it right away, but over time you will.

When you forgive, you have healed the energy between you and the one forgiven. Don't be surprised if you get phone calls out of the blue or Facebook messages from long-lost loved ones or old friends you have officially forgiven. I have! It's as if people know on some level that you have forgiven them, and that they feel better as well. Holding grudges is exhausting; it takes an enormous amount of energy to do so. You might not realize how much baggage you carry day in and day out, but believe me, you want to travel light in life. Forgiveness is a huge step toward attaining this lightness.

I have found that forgiving myself has been much harder than forgiving Kevin, the man from whom I contracted herpes. Many of you might also find this to be the case because we are often the hardest on ourselves. It's not that we consciously chose to be infected with an STD, but somehow we think it's our fault for not knowing any better or for not trusting our instincts about a certain person. Each situation is unique, and some paths that have led you to this journey have been gut-wrenching. Maybe a trusted partner transmitted the virus to you and did so without revealing his or her STD status. Maybe you got it while you were being violated. Have you considered that the person who infected you may have done it unknowingly? Most people who have STDs don't know it, nor do they report any symptoms.

Regardless of the circumstances, forgiveness is the greatest path to freedom. It is also, in my opinion, one of the hardest things to do in life. I am typically not one to hold grudges, but the true surrender necessary to forgive at the deepest of levels requires some difficult work. But if I can do it, so can you! When I practice forgiveness, I feel more in touch with the love I have for humanity and the realization that we are all here, doing the very best we can.

Each and every day we are alive provides us numerous opportunities to practice forgiveness. Just a few weeks ago I came across a YouTube video in which a group of men were apologizing for the atrocities that men have historically committed to women. These men wanted to be part of the solution, encouraging women to lay down our weapons. Even though these men had not been a part of the atrocities, they were, in essence, asking forgiveness for the whole of the male race. Although my husband did not understand why they would apologize for something they had not done, I totally understood where they were coming from, and was moved by their loving gesture.

An STD diagnosis can serve as an amazing teacher of forgiveness. To start, you must forgive yourself and forgive the person who infected you. Every human emotion has a certain energy associated with it, and anger, frustration, and shame are the lowest of energies. To better understand how emotions are linked to energies, think of someone you love giving you a great big hug. How do you feel even when you think about this? Does it bring a smile to your face? Do you feel all warm and fuzzy? Does it lift your spirits or dampen them? Now think of the day you were diagnosed with herpes. Did your shoulders slump? Did you feel heavier? What did the muscles in your face do? Your physical response should clue you into the energy of these events.

The higher your energy state, the more primed you will be for health and healing. Long-standing states of depression, shame, and anger have been linked to symptoms of disease, whereas higher states of joy, love, forgiveness, and peace have been linked to well-being.

I now invite you to begin linking your emotional state with your propensity for healing. If every time you have to have "the Talk" or you have symptoms of your infection, you are cursing up a storm at the person who gave it to you, it's just a matter of time before your symptoms worsen. This burning anger can literally be felt in the tissues of your body. In the end, you will be the one who suffers, not the person who gave you herpes. If you can forgive, then you will set the stage for a deeper level of healing and well-being. Practice, practice, and then practice some more. Forgiveness will set you free!

Forgiving the Unforgivable

The first year of chiropractic school was trying, but extremely fulfilling for me. We nearly lost my grandmother to lung cancer, and at the same time, I witnessed the power of alternative medicine heal someone near and dear to me. My personal life was a bit rocky as I struggled once and for all to finally break things off with Jack, my boyfriend at the time. It was clear to me that he was very manipulative and controlling, but I just couldn't shake him from my life. One minute he would have me screaming to the top of my lungs, and the next minute he would make me feel like all was well in my world.

I will say that in some ways, those who bring us the greatest struggle can also be our greatest teachers. Jack was an angel in that he played a pivotal role in my reclaiming my childhood from sexual abuse. With his help and inroads with the FBI, I was able to bring a pedophile, one of my junior-high teachers, to justice. I debated for several months whether or not to reveal my story to the authorities. My decision to go for it came after a young girl sat next to me on a plane ride home from Puerto Rico.

I had told Jack everything I could remember about the abuse. During a separate conversation, when this little girl told me she was thirteen, I realized that I was her same age when the abuse began. I remember looking out the window of the plane, crying, because I saw my youth and vulnerability in her. Up until that time, I had disconnected to the point that I'd thought I was much older than I was when it all began.

Many other girls came forward while this sex offender was on trial. The outcome of removing him from the school system and alerting the public to his offense allowed me to move forward in my journey toward wholeness. I was motivated to stop the cycle of abuse, and to that end, I was successful. Jack played the hero archetype to a T, but as I got stronger, my need for him waned with each passing day.

I have found that many sufferers of STDs also have had a history of sexual abuse. Many people begin to shun and ignore and maybe even hate their sexual selves because of the pain of association. But it's not your fault you contracted an STD. I believe that the energy of shame is directly linked to both STDs and sexual abuse, and it is not surprising that both trigger similar feelings. When people disconnect from their sexual selves, their bodies will eventually manifest disease and imbalance.

In isolation, our reproductive system will eventually shout out to be heard. Emotions are meant to be expressed, but when we stuff them and ignore them, the stuck energy becomes toxic. This might show up as breast or prostate cancer, infertility, or any number of reproductive health challenges. Remember, disease symptoms are always signposts of something out of balance. An emotional imbalance is just as detrimental to our health as a physical imbalance.

It took me a long time to realize that the shame of having herpes was linked to the shame I associated with being abused. Healing those unintegrated aspects of my past did not happen overnight. If you, too, have experienced abuse, I encourage you to seek the counseling and support you need so that you can heal and become a healthy, vibrant sexual being. Don't sabotage your own health or emotional well-being.

Maybe you have developed other self-sabotaging tendencies, like turning to drugs, alcohol, or food to deaden the pain. If so, your time is now. Take your power back! If you have not done the emotional work necessary to address any violations of your first and second chakras (energy centers found at the base of your spine and into your pelvis), healing an incurable STD will be challenging. STDs can create a subconscious reminder of old, emotionally charged wounds. You have the ability to discover peace and love in these areas of your body. Heck, you might even fall in love with yourself!

You must learn to forgive yourself, any past abusers, and the person who gave you herpes. This is the only path I know that is certain to give you the peace and healing you're looking for. If your STD diagnosis brings up old memories of abuse that have never been addressed, seek help and support. Your ability to heal is directly related to your ability to forgive yourself and others. An STD diagnosis can teach you radical love and compassion for yourself and your body. Choose compassion today!

You must learn to embrace your whole self, and this includes everything you are. No one is perfect, and once you realize this, you can allow your armor to soften. If you want to heal, you have to get your flashlight out and shine a bright light on the monster under the bed.

Our shadows will no longer take charge of our lives once we can acknowledge them. They lose nearly all their charge and power when we can begin to dialogue with them. If your genitals feel sad, don't suppress it. The sadness might run deeper than your infection. Maybe you have felt violated in the past, not just physically, but emotionally. Be compassionate and curious when dialoguing with your body. My paths of healing from sexual abuse and herpes were similar in that both taught me to embrace the feminine and to yield to my inner needs and callings. All of the answers to healing come from within.

An Exercise of Forgiveness

The beauty of this forgiveness exercise is that it does not have to be implemented in person. In fact, the person you are forgiving could be on the other side of the world. I learned this process from my Qigong instructor, and over the years I have adapted it to become my own. It is an exercise based on a principle in energy medicine called "cord cutting." The idea of cord cutting is that you are connected to everyone in your life by energetic cords. The first cord is the physical umbilical chord between you and your mother. Since your birth, you have developed thousands and thousands of energetic cords that attach you to loved ones, friends, coworkers, family members...the list goes on and on. It is an energetic imprint of sorts that determines how you interact with one another.

When a cord is based on negative feelings, it no longer serves you and actually drains you of energy. This is the case when you are harboring negative feelings toward the person who gave you herpes. Every time you have an outbreak, not only are you integrating your emotions about herpes, but you are also expending energy being angry, vengeful, or even hateful. This loss of energy in your system is actually further sabotaging your own ability to heal. Healing takes energy, and at the end of the day, you want to have extra energy to heal, especially while you sleep.

As such, you might want to use this as a meditation before going to bed. This is the same meditation I use when I need to forgive anyone about anything. Have you forgiven your parents for not being perfect? Have you forgiven a childhood bully? What about a sibling you are currently not talking to? Whoever it might be, know that you do not need to speak with them in person. I have even had people take the time to forgive a deceased loved one. Start with the person who gave you herpes and go from there! Free yourself from the things that bind you!

Set aside fifteen minutes where you will not be bothered by anybody or anything. Create a sacred space for yourself in an area of your home where you feel most at ease. Be sure to wear comfortable clothing. Turn off your cell phone, computer, and TV, and remove any distractions from your immediate surroundings. Light some candles, and set an intention for peace.

Sit on some pillows with your back straight. If this is not comfortable, you can modify your position by sitting upright on a chair or couch. Close your eyes and take a deep breath. It is important to breathe through your nose. Feel your breath move all the way down to your belly. Place your hands on your belly and feel your belly expand with the in breath and deflate with the out breath.

When you feel that your mind has settled and you are experiencing ease, bring your attention to your third chakra, residing a couple of inches above your belly button. By breathing into this place you are igniting your power.

Imagine a bubble of vibrant white light surrounding your entire being. Visualize that the person who gave you herpes is sitting across from you. Surround him/her with a separate bubble of vibrant white light.

Imagine a cord that extends from your belly to his/her belly, connecting you both. Do not be surprised if you also feel some energetic chords tapping into other areas of your body. Thank this person for all of the lessons you have learned from him/her, and say out loud, "(Person's Name), I forgive you." Repeat this aloud several times until you feel it is no longer time to do so. If tears come, allow them. This is all part of the healing process.

Imagine yourself cutting the cord that binds you with a pair of imaginary scissors. Allow your end of the cord to recoil back into you as the other end of the cord recoils back into the other person. Come back to your breath. When you feel complete, allow the image of the other person to vanish.

Spend a few more minutes being conscious of your breath and the brilliant light that surrounds you. You are a radiant beam of light and love.

FOUR

Cultivating A Healing Perspective, Intuition, and Chakra Healing

The Traveler, the Prisoner, and the Learner

Most of the shadows of life are caused by standing in our own sunshine.

—RALPH WALDO EMERSON

Learning to live with herpes is not necessarily an easy road, but your perspective on it is everything. Early on, I knew that herpes must be here as a teacher for me, so that I could then teach others. This might seem radical if you have just been diagnosed, but keep in mind that I am the eternal optimist. Lesson number one:

The turnaround from victim to victor can happen almost instantaneously with a change in perspective.

You have the power to create the outcome of any event in your life by the way you choose to respond to it. By becoming a prisoner, traveler, or learner, you actively choose the type of person you become in any given event. The prisoner chooses to disengage, break down, and hold the perspective of victim. She is a prisoner of her own life. The traveler, on the other hand, approaches life and its events as if she has no control over them. Although she doesn't feel sorry for herself, she just moves with the changing tide. The traveler is extremely passive in her response to adversity. The last role in this play of life is the learner, who is the captain of her own ship. This champion chooses to rise above adversity and to learn from her experiences. She searches for the gifts that her greatest challenges bring. Choose to be a learner and you are set free. When we can come from the perspective of the learner, we are set free from the role of victim and we actively engage in what life throws our way. What role do *you* want to play in life?

A Learner in Action

When I was seventeen years old, I spent a summer in Portugal as a foreign-exchange student in a home-stay program. Although I did not speak a word of Portuguese, I chose the country purely on the basis of my AFS (American Field Service) counselor's desire to send a student from our high school there. When I submitted my application, all of the more popular countries were already taken. So, being the adventurer I was, I agreed to be the guinea-pig kid and head to Portugal.

Flipping through photos of beaches, castles, and hillside towns, I thought my summer was sure to be an adventure of a lifetime. Little did I know, the family I was to stay with did not really want me there. The older daughter, a successful lawyer living an hour away in Lisbon, thought that an American foreign exchange student would be the perfect solution for her painfully shy teenage sister who was still living at home. After I arrived, it was clear that the younger daughter, my new "sister," thought otherwise.

My Portuguese family was far from the one I imagined in my dreams. Where shall I begin my laundry list of disappointments? Their small home smelled of rotten fish; the kitchen was stacked to the gills with filthy dishes; the TV blared soap operas and *Sesame Street* all day; and the damned cat sprayed through the whole house, careful not to miss my flea-infested bed! The mother seemed truly indifferent to my needs or whereabouts. Since she did not speak a lick of English and I knew nothing of the Portuguese language, our only communication throughout the summer was her ever-present scowl and some "blah, blah, blah," as she waved her hands in frustration. The daughter was my only potential saving grace, but her English was extremely limited, and she preferred to knit rather than talk to me.

During my first few days there, I cried myself to sleep, questioning how I would ever make it through the eight weeks of my summer stay. After several depressing days, I decided to explore the areas outside of my neighborhood and take a bus ride into the beautiful fishing village of Cascais. A crumpled and worn bus schedule and my handy English-to-Portuguese dictionary were my only companions. The hell that I was living in could be no worse than getting lost and sleeping on the street, I thought. What if I *did* get lost and couldn't find my way home? I was ready to take the risk, even though I questioned how long it would take before my family even noticed me missing.

With a bit of trepidation and excitement, I rode a Saturday bus full of locals and their chickens into town. "I'm an American!" was written all over my youthful face. I sat quietly, rubbernecked every passing sign, and memorized the landscape for my return home. Questioning my every move, I pulled the wire to get off the bus. The bell rang, and I was off on a grand adventure to find the beach. Thank God for the Portuguese signs with pictures on them! A picture is worth a thousand words, especially when you are navigating your way through foreign lands. With a little bit of intuition, common sense, and a few gestures and interactions with the local people, I found my way to the beach.

The beach was not as pristine and jaw dropping as I had hoped, but the colorful fishing boats bobbing in the distance were picturesque. Several thousand miles from home, I stretched out my towel and surrendered to the warmth of the sun. After a few dips in the water and a cold soda to quench my thirst, I met a lovely family vacationing from Germany. I struck up a great conversation with their daughter, who was about my age. Our kindred spirits immediately connected, and she became my first real friend on my journey. As the sun's rays were softening and the day was coming to an end, I brushed the sand off of my feet, exchanged phone numbers with my new friend, and headed for a late-afternoon coffee.

While sipping coffee, overlooking the beach and steadying my journal on an uneven two-top table, I met Guillermo. That coffee turned into many as Guillermo became my best friend, translator, and tour guide for the rest of the summer.

After I met Guillermo (Portuguese for William), gone were my days of loneliness and regret. My days were now filled with fun. Each morning, several hours after the sunrise, Guillermo and I would zoom off on his moped to explore castles and secluded beaches. To think that our relationship was totally platonic was pretty amazing. He was smart, handsome, and knew how to show a girl a good time without *ever* making any advances. We logged many miles on his moped that summer; it was our passport to adventure. On any given day, a posse of his friends would join us on their mopeds. Nights were spent laughing, dancing, playing pool, and hanging out in coffee shops and nightclubs. I was able to have a firsthand experience of how coffee shops can become a center for community and conversation. This was before Starbucks and personal computers infiltrated the world.

My Portuguese friends accepted me into their circle of fun, as if I had always been a part of their group. It no longer mattered to me what was going on at home. It became merely a place to lay my head at night. I adopted my own family for the summer—my friends. It is through them that I learned about the history and the culture of Portugal. Needless to say, I spent very little time with my Portuguese family that summer, and I can honestly say that I had the time of my life. I left very tan, with sun-bleached hair, a pocketful of Portuguese words, and a lifetime of stories to tell.

This story represents all the roles of prisoner, traveler, and learner. The prisoner would have never left the house. She would have cried herself to sleep every night, blaming her AFS counselor and wishing she had never left the US. The traveler would have hunkered down in the local hood, maybe learning a few words, hanging out in the local cafe and counting down the days until the summer ended. After doing a bit of the first two, I *chose* to be the learner. I reached out beyond my comfort zone and explored a foreign country, with my arms outstretched and my heart leading me with blind faith. I submerged myself in the language and the culture, and as a result gained a new skill set for life. To this day, I feel confident that I can figure my way around any situation in just about any country. In many ways, you are never really lost if there are people around you who can guide you, even if you don't speak their language!

You, too, can decide how you will respond to your herpes. If you choose to be the prisoner, your life will probably be lonely and depressing. Choose to be the traveler, and you might never receive the blessings that herpes is here to bestow upon you. You might never commit to a life of health and happiness. By becoming a learner, you begin to learn and practice forgiveness and deepen your level of self-love, using affirmations and speaking your truth. You believe in your capacity to heal herpes and know that you are deserving of love. By becoming the learner, you have an excellent shot at totally altering your path in life. You, too, can create your reality. You can choose love, health, and happiness. Decide right now which path you choose to take, for your life will never be the same.

Victim and Victor

Jack Canfield, coauthor of *Chicken Soup for the Soul*, taught me a very important lesson over a decade ago. He explained how we have the ability to overcome any past event by changing our perspective on it. Much like choosing to become a learner, you can also choose to be the victor over your herpes. Many people who are diagnosed with herpes start out feeling victimized by their infection. This is normal, but it becomes a problem if they remain in "victim mode" for their entire lives. To feel victimized is part of the healing journey. I certainly started there, and it took me several years to move toward and eventually embody the victor.

As you gain personal strength and emotional rebalancing, you, too, can become a victor. To be a victor means that you know you are more than your herpes and have powerfully decided to relate to the virus and your symptoms in a positive light. As you begin to take "response-ability"—being conscious of your ability to form a positive response for every event in your life—you will move from victim to victor. Are great world leaders victims? Absolutely not! Even if you have no desire to be a great world leader, choose to be the great leader of your own life. Take challenges, and like a great alchemist, turn tragedy into triumph!

Dig deep and rediscover your inner strengths. Educating yourself about herpes is one of the best things you can do to regain some emotional balancing and control. If you are confused, it is very challenging to move forward. When we are confused, we are disempowered. Educating yourself about your new diagnosis will bring a new level of clarity. So, how do you know if you are in victim mode or victor mode? Use the lists below to determine your perspective.

When you choose to identify with the role of the victim, you:
- Believe you are unlovable, dirty or shameful
- Begin to self-sabotage by overeating, drinking, and/or using drugs
- Turn to a life of celibacy, even though this is not your true desire
- Harbor anger and vengeful thoughts toward the person who gave you herpes
- Turn a blind eye and pretend that you don't have it, infecting others along the way
- Keep herpes a secret and shun all levels of intimacy
- Ignore your own power to heal
- Choose to remain confused

When you choose to identify with the role of the victor, you:
- Remain open and share your story
- Learn all that you can about the herpes virus and how to manage it in a way that empowers you
- Discover an entire new level of self-love and forgiveness
- Open yourself up to new perspectives of healing
- Become honest and truthful with your intimate partners and take responsible actions
- Get in touch with your inner goddess
- Learn to forgive yourself and others
- Learn how to connect to others on a deeper level
- Begin a journey of transformation
- Empower and inspire others to heal

Drink the Juice of Positive Thinking

Your thoughts and language are incredibly powerful. Who would you be without your negative self-talk? How would you move in the world differently if you perceived yourself as a victor in life instead of a victim? Do you ever listen to how you refer to yourself? Begin to listen to your dialogue. "I'm so stupid…No one will ever love me…I'm so fat." I may not have hit your trigger, but I can almost guarantee that you have some negative dialogue going on. Everybody does this; it is more of a matter of *to what degree*. My husband and I have the kind of relationship in which we acknowledge when one of us has said something that is not serving us. I am so grateful to have him call me out on my BS. If we are to become conscious, enlightened beings, then we need to be mindful of how our emotional state affects our ability to heal.

Healing with Positive Thinking: A Top-Ten List to Transform Your Life

1. Place a rubber band around your wrist for a week and snap yourself silly whenever you say something negative about yourself or someone else. Once you make yourself conscious of the frequency with which you say negative things, you may be shocked.
2. Each time you say something negative, say, "Cancel that," and replace it with a positive thought.
3. Be playful with higher states of consciousness, and experiment with them in your daily life. For example, I have playfully experimented with smiling while I do yoga to access higher states of joy. I imagine even my little toes feeling joy and the perfection of the universe.
4. If you are feeling one of the lower vibrations, a vibration of sadness or shame, feel into it, and then try to think of something you could do to raise your vibration to joy, love, or peace, even one step higher. Think of one thing you are grateful for.
5. Move your body! It has an immediate impact on your feelings. Movement will fire off input to your brain and will immediately change the state of your brain. Do some jumping jacks or punch a pillow. Whatever you feel inspired to do, just move!
6. Surround yourself with positive-thinking people.
7. Remove yourself from everyday Scrooges. You will be amazed how much your social environment can impact you.
8. Be aware of the negativity that surrounds you, and begin to make some changes.
9. Remember that you are the only one who can allow others to make you feel small.

10. Stop reading the paper and watching the news. It's nothing but negativity! Instead of listening to NPR and world affairs, pop some self-help gurus like Tony Robbins or Wayne Dyer into your audio cue.

Once you become more conscious of these higher states, you will want to be in them all the time. Bliss and pure consciousness are more addictive than *any* drug, and these higher states will directly impact your body's ability to heal. Your emotions are real, and they greatly impact your everyday life.

You Can Heal Your Life: Louise Hay's Story

The movie *You Can Heal Your Life* is based on Louise Hay's work as a self-help pioneer. She is the kind of woman who entered her eighties convinced that it would be her best decade yet! Hay has built an empire based on positive thinking and affirmations as tools for transforming one's life. I am in awe of her radiant, pioneering spirit and the inspiring contributions she has made to society through her books, workshops, and the launch of Hay House, Inc. *You Can Heal Your Life* is a documentary featuring a stellar cast of self-help gurus that includes Wayne Dyer, Jerry and Ester Hicks, Gay Hendrix, Doreen Virtue, and Louise Hay. In it, each shares his or her unique life challenges, which sometimes included physical, emotional, or sexual abuse.

At the age of fifteen, Hay left her abusive home and set out to create a new reality for herself. She recollects leaving her atrocious home environment as a high school dropout with limited social skills. All she knew was that in order to change her life, she had to remove herself, and later her mother, from a toxic environment. She began working at five-and-dime establishments, became a model in New York, and eventually discovered healing through metaphysical practices. These practices and life experiences lead her to a career as a therapist, best-selling author, and workshop leader. She is known for healing herself of vaginal cancer by using only the healing tools she had learned and taught over the years. In her opinion, her cancer was directly linked to the shame and guilt of being repeatedly raped as a child, much like how I believe that STIs (sexually transmitted infections) are linked to our subconscious feelings of shame. Her success in healing herself was the last step she needed to embody her teachings and practices.

Louise Hay's story epitomizes our ability to turn our greatest challenges in life to our greatest gifts. Other great leaders in the self-help world have also used their stories of triumph as fuel to make the world a better place. Take the time to learn more about people you admire, like Wayne Dyer, the orphan of an alcoholic; Debbie Ford, a reformed drug user; and Oprah Winfrey, a victim of sexual abuse. There is no shortage of inspiring people who light up the world, despite the fact that they came from very challenging pasts. Allow these leaders to be your source of inspiration as you triumph over your diagnosis of herpes.

We can learn a great deal from Hay as we begin to use the techniques and practices she taught. During the 1980s, Louise Hay began working with the HIV/AIDS population in San Francisco, assisting them in developing a positive attitude and approach to their disease. A client of hers had requested that she start a support group for gay men with HIV/AIDS in the Bay Area. What started out as a meeting of just six men eventually turned into a weekly gathering of eight hundred men and the beginnings of The Hay Foundation. This was groundbreaking at a time when no one felt safe talking about HIV/AIDS and very few people had even heard of positive affirmations or how negative mental thought patterns could aid a disease. Central to her therapy were three main things:

- How to dissolve resentment
- Forgiveness
- Self-love

Sound familiar? These are the same things that she needed to learn on a cellular level in healing vaginal cancer and the same things I have worked through to manage herpes.

Adapting these concepts above, through meditations, affirmations, singing, and public sharing, the men began to sleep better and feel better about themselves. My guess is that they also began to experience some radical healing. Public acceptance of HIV/AIDS has grown leaps and bounds over the years, but there is still work to be done. Herpes is much different in that it is not deadly, but there are several parallels here to bare in mind. Both conditions embody the emotions of shame, guilt, anger, and resentment. These diseases are intimately entwined with our sexual psyche, and they carry with them a social stigma. When you are diagnosed with either condition, it is very easy to think of your body as a battlefield and to think that your body is your enemy. Herpes is not the enemy, nor is your body.

In her book *HealYour Body*, Louise Hay lists dozens of diseases or discomforts with a probable cause and affirmation for healing. She explains how all ailments are directly linked to some negative thought pattern. In order to heal the ailment, you must create a positive thought pattern that can be verbalized in a healing affirmation. For example, Louise Hay states that if your problem is getting cold sores, the probable cause is harboring angry words and having fear of expressing them. The new positive thought pattern could be an affirmation like, "I only create peaceful experiences because I love myself. All is well." This affirmation would be repeated several times a day. Genital herpes is another ailment she discusses. She explains that this problem is rooted in sexual guilt, experiencing public shame, and rejection of the genitals. In order to overcome this you might say, "I am beautiful, perfect, and normal. I rejoice in my sexuality and my own unique body."

My experience in sharing these affirmations with other women who have herpes has been a very powerful and eye-opening exercise. Whether it's genital herpes or a toothache, many women have been able to associate the probable cause from something in their past. If the above statements do not ring true for you, feel free to disregard them, discover your own most probable cause, and create new positive thought patterns or affirmations. You may have insight if you allow yourself the space for reflection or meditation. When you do find something that resonates with you, commit to stating the new thought pattern/affirmation several times a day. It is especially powerful to state it first thing in the morning and right before bed while your ego is a bit sleepy and less able to override the new thought.

Begin to Cancel Out Negative Self-Talk with Positive Declarations

You have the choice to embrace your day. Put positive intentions into it and move with the direction life wants you to go. You will be amazed at how things shift for you when you start your day with positive intentions. When you get clear and present with your desires, you attract them into your life. Here are some affirmations below, but get creative and write out ones that serve you best!

Affirmations

Life comes to me easily and effortlessly.

I am happy, healthy, and whole.

I am a beautiful and brilliant woman.

I am a magnet for love.

I love all of who I am.

Money comes to me easily and effortlessly.

I am in the FLOW.

I am beautiful, bountiful, and blissful.

I forgive all past experiences.

I love you very much, (your name).

All is well; I am safe.

I am completely lovable.

I love and approve of myself.

My body now restores itself to its natural state of health.

I give and receive love every day.

I am safe to be me.

I speak my truth.

I love my body.

All is provided for now.

My intuition is a powerful guide.

Print or write your affirmations out and place them on your bathroom mirror! Say them with enthusiasm, even if you don't feel them in your body yet. If you make your own affirmation, use any verbs in the present tense as if they are true now. For example, you would never say, "I will be the best mother in the world." You would instead say, "I am the best mother in the world." Use your emotions as a guideline to where you currently are. Over time, you will embody these thoughts as truth. It's OK if you start out just going through the motions. Eventually, your emotions will catch up with the higher vibration of these powerful words.

Being in the Flow

When we move with the direction life wants to move us, instead of fighting against the universal current, we are experiencing the flow of life. We are supported and can float effortlessly. Flow is experiencing the truth of your life. It is at the center of life's movement. It is from that place that the brain, body, and life force are in clear communication. In other words, when you are in flow, you take full response-ability for your life.

Our desire to create an abundant life comes from a deeply seeded belief that our thoughts create our reality and that the universe is a safe and inviting place to live. This is a power that we all have, and it manifests when we tap into this movement of life.

Water is a great metaphor for flow, for it moves to the area of least resistance. Fundamentally, when we are in flow, we have the ability to respond to our environment with great ease. We all know what it is like to be in that place of flow, when there is grace in just about everything that happens. When we chose to move with life, life is easy. Are you allowing your internal flow to guide you, or are you like a salmon, swimming upstream to spawn and take your last breath? In order to be in this place, you must be present to the external cues in your life and respond with internal knowing, or your intuition. This might be a leap of faith for you, but stay with me.

You can begin to invite flow into your life through intention and affirmation from the time your eyes open up in the morning to the time your head hits the pillow at night. I might wake up and think, "I would love a large glass of water," and out into the universe my thought goes. Before I have time to go downstairs and get some water, my husband lovingly hands me a glass. This is flow! When you think, "I would love a front-row parking spot at the movie theater tonight," and as you pull up to the theater, rock-star parking appears—this is flow. Consciously and continuously bless your day with positive intentions.

If you want to live an extraordinary life that is filled with blessings and bliss, you must learn to better respond to your internal and external cues. This is the very reason that I am constantly seeking silence and higher states of consciousness, where I am able to intuit what I need to be doing in each and every moment. Reducing stress, eating correctly, exercising, detoxing, meditation, and positive self-talk are just a few of the things you can be doing to raise your vibration so that you can consciously connect to the gifts of life.

Using Intuition to Heal Your Herpes

*If you heed to your inner callings, you will find yourself
in a world where you dance in perfect timing.*

Have you ever had the feeling that your mother was going to call you and then she did, or you heard your husband's car in your driveway and looked out of your window only to see that nothing was there, and then ten minutes later he walked through the door? That is, in a sense, an aspect of intuition—an internal knowing based on your senses.

When you are on the right path in life, things truly do flow, and you feel as though you are divinely guided. Life begins to show you signposts for your next move. It is as if the lens through which you view your life becomes a bit clearer. All of the smudges and dirt are wiped clear, and you can begin to see through a veil that appeared to separate you from spirit. I know that you have experienced some level of flow and intuition at some point in your life. Intuition might come to you in the form of a thought, dream, feeling, smell, sound, or any number of ways. I personally feel energy moving in my lips and teeth when I am working on someone or am receiving healing. It is my internal cue that the energy in my environment is shifting.

When you are on a healing path, you will begin to notice more and more synchronicities. Begin to listen to your inner callings as they guide you in life. I have always said that if I hear or see something more than three times, then I should probably being paying close attention to what it's trying to tell me. Part of your journey in healing herpes is to listen to your inner guru. What herbs, foods, or practitioners are you drawn to? Have you had any dreams that might offer some guidance? When you are in the flow of life, you will know exactly what to do.

Forms of Intuition

Just trust yourself. Then you will know how to live.

—GOETHE

Intuition is such a juicy topic for me to write about because it evokes the elements of mystery and magic. It is something that everyone has been gifted with but few tap into. Intuition is an invaluable guide and keeps you from harm's way. Intuition and our senses give us the tools to respond to our ever-changing environment. Although we are quite knowledgeable regarding our five senses of sight, smell, touch, hearing, and taste, there is a sixth sense, a sense that most often goes unexplored. This sixth sense is the invaluable faculty of intuition. For most of us, it is challenging to find the right vocabulary to explain the feeling of intuition. I have heard people say, "I can't quite put my finger on it, but I have a feeling that…" It is often defined as a quick insight, a sense of knowing, and independent of any reasoning process.

One of the greatest examples of intuition was found in the behavior of animals before the waves of the 2004 South East Asian Tsunami hit the coasts of Sri Lanka. Approximately 275,000 people died in this devastating event that affected over eleven countries, and yet relatively few animals were killed in this tragedy. Why? Wildlife experts believe that the animals knew the tsunami was coming. Eyewitnesses saw both domestic and wild animals seeking higher ground and shelter. Evidently, the animals were responding to what we might call a sixth sense. Haven't you ever had an experience and later thought, "If only I had listened to my gut feeling or intuition?" Some doctors believe that there exists a "second brain" of sorts in your gut, so in this case, a gut feeling to seek higher ground would have saved your life. To be in the flow is to be receptive to all of life.

I believe that people are able to access their intuition when they actively respond to both their internal and external environments. It is so important that we begin to notice the signposts that surround us in life. Sometimes these will be gentle nudges, and other times they will be glaringly obvious. This heightened form of awareness can come in many forms. Below is a list of ways that your body might guide you.

Visual

Visual intuition involves seeing something beyond the perception of the physical eye. This might include seeing auras (colored energy surrounding people, plants, or animals), angels, people, animals, and other subjects that are taken out of usual context. When you see these things, they are not in physical form. This can also include seeing something repeatedly that might be a symbol for something in your life.

Example: You are considering adopting a puppy from your local humane society. This puppy is a rare breed that you know very little about. All in the same day, you see someone walking this same breed down your street, you see one on TV, and your friend mentions this breed in her daily blog. Should you adopt? I think so!

Auditory

You may hear an inner voice speaking to you or hear a sound that did not actually occur or that reminds you of something.

Example: You are driving home from work, and you hear an inner voice telling you to go home using an alternative route. You follow this guidance, and on the evening news you discover that there was a major accident on your normal commute home. You might have been stuck in traffic for hours, or you might have been involved in the accident. Please listen to these inner callings, as they can be telling you something very important.

Taste/Smell

A taste or smell may trigger a thought or create an experience that you feel has happened before.

Example: You walk into a store and smell a unique perfume that only your grandmother wears. You have not talked to her for several months. You decide to call her and discover she is sick and not doing well. You now know why you were drawn to call her, for your call comforted her, and the sound of your voice lifted her spirits.

Kinesthetic/Gut Feeling

This is the experience of altered feelings or sensations in your body. It could be a number of things, from a knot in your stomach to warmth in your chest, ultimately defining what intuition is. Everybody is unique, so it's important to pay attention to your own body and what it is trying to tell you.

Example: You are actively looking for a new massage therapist. When you come home from a long workday, you notice a hanger on your door. It is a coupon to receive twenty dollars off your first massage with a specific company. As you read the coupon, you feel your heart open up a bit and an immediate urge to make an appointment. Should you call? Absolutely!

Dreams

Some people dream in symbols while others have foreshadowing events happen in their dreams. A dream can be a window into the soul's desire or can serve to solve some quandary. If you have a question in life and need some guidance, clearly ask for what you want and use the dream state or meditative state to receive answers. I like to do this right before bed when I am troubled by something. I ask that my dreams show me how to overcome a problem or allow me to have insight into that which is troubling me.

Example: Many of our presidents and leaders have had foreshadowing dreams. Abraham Lincoln dreamed of his assassination before it happened and shared this dream with his wife.

Synchronicities

Timing is everything in life, right? Synchronicities are interpreting the random experiences you have in life so that they are able to lead you in the right direction. This somewhat chaotic world does, in fact, have patterns that can be noticed when you are paying attention. External signs and clues often let you know that you are on the right path. This is not intuition, but is essentially just another instrument that can work as a guide.

Example: Let's say you have always dreamed of having your own bakery—a wedding cake specialty shop. Up until now, your full-time job has stood in the way of your dreams. One day you show up to work only to discover that you have been laid off, even though you have served the company for over thirty years. Free to pursue your dreams, you start looking for a kitchen space to lease, and on the exact same day, a friend calls you and tells you that she would like to commission you to bake her wedding cake. Happenstance? I think not!

The older I get, the more I rely on my intuition as a guiding force in my life. It is the difference between moving with the current of life or moving against it. While some enjoy the challenge of swimming upstream, I prefer to go with the flow. When something doesn't quite feel right or is seemingly very hard, this usually signifies that I am moving against the current of my life. I believe that on a very primitive level we are wired for intuition to keep us from harm.

For many thousands of years, humans, just as animals have done, have been able to psychically intuit many events: a tiger approaching the village in which we live, knowing a storm is approaching, or feeling that our child is in danger before the events occur. As we move throughout the generations and into an environment surrounded by technology rather than nature, we become less aware of ourselves and our natural environment, taking us further away from the ability to connect to our intuition. While we might not be in as much physical danger as we once were, we could all still benefit from tapping into our intuition. Think of your intuition as a muscle that needs to be worked on a daily basis. Do your intuition "push-ups" by checking in with your intuitive feelings on a regular basis.

So, how do you reconnect with your intuition muscle? Practicing the ability to tap into awareness and building trust with yourself is the first thing that will help you connect with your intuition muscle. Intuition is not based on knowledge, but rather on something that is often intangible. The mind will constantly creep in and steer you away from feeling to thinking, and it is your job to keep the "monkey mind" at bay so that you are able to fully feel your body and the messages it's giving you. If the "thinking" mind is engaged, it will almost always alter the outcome of what you are trying to intuit.

For example, let us say that your best friend is pregnant, and she has all of the symptoms that might be associated with having a girl. If you want to see if you can intuit the sex of her baby, you will need to clear you mind and ignore the "facts" at hand. If you don't clear your mind first, then your mind will probably weigh the scales toward it being a girl. This is a very important lesson when you are learning how to "feel into" a pressing question or challenge. Do not give your mind a vote!

If using your intuition is totally foreign to you or if you don't trust yourself, here is an exercise to clear the mind. This will allow you to become centered and to access your higher truth.

The Elevator Exercise: Getting Out of Your Head and into Your Body

This is a great exercise to move the energy from your mind and into your body. It is much easier to access your intuition when you can ground the frantic, scattered energy of the mind and move into the slower-paced, more centered "mind" of the body. If you have a question that you need guidance on, do this exercise first as preparation.

Sit in a comfortable position. Close your eyes and pay attention to your in and out breaths. Allow the breath to become deeper and fuller. Let your stress and worries be released with the out breath. Imagine an elevator that sits in the middle of your brain. It is full of all of your thoughts and begins to descend down your entire body. As the elevator descends, follow it slowly with your inner eye. Relax all of the muscles from your brain, neck, and shoulders. Continue to breathe into your chest and heart. Bring your breath into your stomach, pelvis, upper thighs, knees, and finally into your lower legs and feet. Feel your entire body fully relax. Go slowly; at each level of your body, acknowledge that area with breath and ease. Open your eyes when you are able to bring your full attention from the mind into the body. Your body is the place where you fully access your intuition.

Now that you have done the elevator exercise, you are ready to sit with a question that you have been pondering. Start with something easy, like what you want for dinner. Consider that whatever food choice comes to mind might contain certain nutrients your body is deficient in. Always trust the first thing that comes to mind. This is no different than taking a multiple-choice test and knowing that your initial response was most likely the right choice for you. My teachers always warned my classmates and me about changing our answers at the end of an exam. Your intuition is no different. Do not allow your monkey mind to give its opinion. As you begin to practice, your intuition muscle will get stronger and stronger. Release any attachment to the outcome of your inner questions, and always follow through with the answers. If it is a yes-or-no question and it gives you the opportunity to act out the answer, do it! This will build your inner trust. The more you practice, the stronger you will become.

Over time you will begin to develop all sorts of inner guidance tools. You might start out with just a feeling in your gut and eventually develop the ability to track your dreams or listen to an inner voice. Once you begin to trust yourself, you will be far more able to follow the flow of life. If your intuition guides you to what appears to be an unfavorable outcome, ask yourself if there were any hidden treasures. For example, let's say that you are beginning to date someone and you think he is the one. All of your intuitive flags are flying. Two weeks later you learn that he is an absolute jerk, so you begin to question your inner tools. After some inward work, you realize that he was the perfect teacher for you for developing patience in your life. Maybe he taught you the attribution of patience, a much-needed lesson in life. In that respect, your intuition guided you to a man who would serve you in a different way than you might have thought. He was still the one, but for a different reason. This is still intuition working at hand.

Use your intuition to guide you during your journey with herpes. This is holistic medicine at its best. Listen to your inner callings when deciding which supplements you wish to try first, when the best time to exercise is, the most peaceful time of day to mediate, and the foods best suited to your unique healing process. Be willing to be guided by an inner knowing. When times get rough, get quiet, do the elevator exercise, and listen to your inner truth.

Healing Herpes through Your Chakras

I believe that clearing out your energy chakras is essential for you to connect to the flow of life. Your energetic body is composed of seven main energy centers, also known as chakras. These chakras resemble water wheels as they spin around and around. The first one lies at the root of your spine, and the seventh one lies at the crown of your head. The third chakra resides around your navel. This is where you give and receive your power.

It is important for all of these chakras to be in balance in order to experience optimal health. When the flow of energy is stuck in these chakras, it can result in blocked energy flow to vital organs and can also affect the way in which we interact with our world. For example, if you have your fourth chakra (heart chakra) restricted, you may develop heart abnormalities or difficulties in finding and maintaining loving relationships. When your second chakra (pelvic chakra) is restricted, you might have challenges with your menses or fertility.

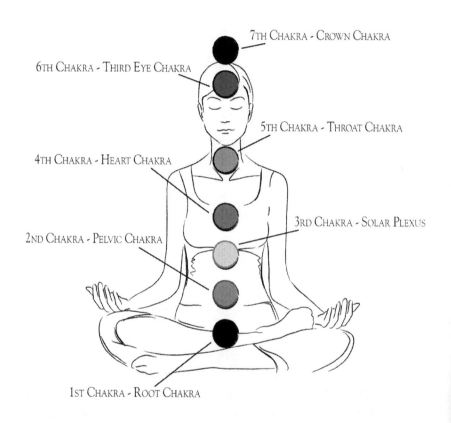

7TH CHAKRA - CROWN CHAKRA

6TH CHAKRA - THIRD EYE CHAKRA

5TH CHAKRA - THROAT CHAKRA

4TH CHAKRA - HEART CHAKRA

3RD CHAKRA - SOLAR PLEXUS

2ND CHAKRA - PELVIC CHAKRA

1ST CHAKRA - ROOT CHAKRA

The Chakras

When you are suffering from genital herpes, your first, second, third, and fourth chakras are directly affected. Herpes tends to close off these areas, and for some, these areas were energetically blocked even years before they got herpes. Either way, I encourage you to begin by clearing any stuck energy in your first and third chakras. As you heal, your fourth chakra will begin to expand as you discover a whole new level of self-love.

There are several ways to open up and clear these chakras. The exercises that follow have the greatest impact on women who have genital herpes. I have met several long-time healing practitioners who have said herpes has allowed them to become much more aware of their energy centers.

First Chakra Clearing Exercise: Your Grounding Cord

Our first chakra is our root chakra, related to elements of survival, including money, shelter, and food. It represents our most primitive human needs. When it is balanced, we feel grounded and effortlessly supported by the universe. People who are not grounded in this way are often a bit more airy, spacy, and noncommittal souls.

The very best way to do this exercise is in a natural setting on solid earth. So, if the outdoors is accessible to you, take advantage of it. Find a comfortable seated position on the ground or in a chair. Close your eyes and begin to take several deep breaths, letting your mind go with each passing breath. Roll your ankles from left to right, straighten your back, and lift your chin off of your chest and expand your heart. Allow your shoulders to drop and your breath to expand. Feel your belly expand with each passing breath. Feel the breath travel all the way down to your tailbone. After you do this several times, feel a root extending from your tailbone into the earth. Pretend you are a thriving oak tree, feeling into your deep root system.

Follow the root as it travels into the ground to the depth of an inch, then a foot, eight feet, one hundred feet, three hundred feet, a mile, one thousand miles, following the root deeper and deeper until it reaches the core of the earth and branches out for miles and miles. Once you feel totally grounded, slowly open your eyes. Gently gaze ahead and allow your breath to return to normal. Slowly move from an inner presence to an outer presence. Wiggle your toes, roll your shoulders, take a deep breath, and slowly reenter your physical world. This practice can take a few minutes or an hour depending on what space you are in, emotionally and physically.

Revitalizing Chakra Three: Call Your Power Back!

Are you totally exhausted and drained at the end of the day? Are there people in your life who zap your energy? Do you give, give, give, and never ask for anything in return? As women, we are natural nurturers, and yet many of us forget to nurture ourselves. This leaves us in a very depleted place where there is no available energy at the end of the day to repair and nourish ourselves.

Our power lies in our third chakra, a couple of inches above our belly button. This is where our mother gave us all of our nourishment when we were still in utero, and some consider it the source of our life force. In the practice of Qigong (a healing and martial art form from ancient China), this area of the body is near the lower *dan tien*. Qigong practitioners stimulate this area to rebuild this energy center and to restore health and well-being.

Imagine your third chakra as being like your wallet. The more money you have in it, the more "buying power" you have for life. As women, we are constantly leaking energy, or "money," from this center throughout the day. Sometimes we leave our wallets wide open so others can grab as much money and power as they need from us. As with any exchange, it takes energy to get energy, and hopefully most of your energetic exchanges in life are equal in value. Unfortunately, it is not uncommon for us to give ourselves away to the point of exhaustion. There are also people out there that some might call energy vampires because they leave us feeling totally depleted and are tuned into our innocence and good nature. Some energy vampires don't actually realize that they zap others of energy. It might be a good idea to see how you feel after meeting with a friend, neighbor, employee, or boss to see where your energy levels are. If you are exhausted after every interaction, you may have identified a potential energy vampire in your life.

At the end of the day, many people are totally unaware of how much energy and power they have leaked. As you go through your day, practice identifying where you may have left a part of your energy or power. Did you leave some in the grocery store when you were angry for someone cutting you off? Did you leave some with your children as they were pushing your buttons and limits? Did you just let your friend dump all of her drama on you, leaving you feeling exhausted? Consciously go through your day, and call all of your energy back to your third chakra. Put your hands on your upper belly and take several deep belly breaths as you call your power back. Refill your bank account! You are the only one who can use your energy, or "money," so having your personalized Ben Franklins scattered throughout your town does nobody any good. Learning to say no is often a skill set that comes along with honoring your third chakra and power center.

The more you call your energy back to your third chakra, the more aware you'll be of noticing what activities and people are taking your energy. You will also notice that you feel more energetic and centered. When you identify any inappropriate boundaries being crossed, know you have the power to speak your truth and compassionately articulate your desire for a shift. At some point, you will no longer need to consciously do this because you will become acutely aware of your energetic exchanges with people. Most importantly, it's vital that you understand this: only when you have respect for yourself will others give you respect.

Healing Chakras One through Four: Breath Is Life

The next time you are around a sleeping infant, observe his or her breathing. See the depth of breath and movement in the body and spine. If you notice carefully, the breath moves in and out of the body like an undulating wave. Watch as the tidal breath comes in and out and in again. It is mesmerizing to observe such peace and perfection.

Now, become aware of your own breath. Do you feel it in your chest? Your midsection? Your belly? Is your spine moving like a tidal wave, gently massaging each and every vertebra and organ? What went wrong? The stress of life. Somewhere along the way, we shut down and became stressed-out, shallow breathers. We began to carry our whole life of trials and tribulations in our tight muscles, organs, and postures of defeat. Think back to the last time you took a conscious breath. How many of these breaths do you think you take a day? One, two, ten? Many of us can't recall taking even one. As Western women, we spend most of our lives sucking our bellies in, rarely breathing deep into our bellies and allowing them to pooch out.

Breathing fully and effortlessly is the gift that God gives us to remain present in our surroundings, but very few people take advantage of this gift on a daily basis. Many meditation practices utilize the breath to get people out of their minds and back into their bodies. When we bring our consciousness to our breath, we become more aware of our body position, muscles, environment, and thoughts, allowing us to tackle what is at hand rather than walking away from it. When our awareness is focused on our breath, the parasympathetic nervous system, our system of "rest and digest" begins to engage. This is the part of the nervous system that we want to tap into!

Most people are living in the "flight or fight" system, the sympathetic nervous system. It is very challenging to heal when we are predominantly in this system. Conscious breath work will assist your body to move into the healing state of the parasympathetic nervous system. This is where stress levels and blood pressure drop, rebuilding the immunity while also detoxifying waste. The more time that you spend in this state, the faster your body will heal both physically and emotionally.

I am a big fan of breath work for reducing stress and facilitating healing. By incorporating the exercise below, you will begin to reacquaint yourself with your root chakra (chakra one), your sexual chakra (chakra two), your power chakra (chakra three), and your heart chakra (chakra four). The energetic placement of our chakras is constantly shifting, so it's best to continuously work on it. How are you to be a brilliant goddess when your chakras are energetically stuck?

I have found that most Western women have no understanding of how to utilize their breath daily as a practice of meditation and healing. The breath is the silent gauge that continuously informs you how you are doing. Are you stressed about an upcoming work project? Are you nervous about your child's first day of school? Are you suppressing feelings of hurt when your partner is late for dinner? If you use your breath as a tool to relax your body, you can almost immediately tell if something is bothering you or if you are fluidly moving through your life in a relaxed way.

Phase One

Lie down on your back. Get comfortable and try to have your head in line with your spine and not raised above your chest and heart. Slowly become aware of your breath. Place your hands on the area of your body that appears to rise and fall with each passing breath. For example, your lower belly or the area around your heart is a good place to start. When you inhale and exhale with intention, your breath will begin to slow down and get deeper into your body. Feel your hands rise and fall. This is your first position.

Visualize the division of your torso into two sections, an upper part (chest) and lower part (belly). These areas relate, respectively, to the fourth chakra (chest) and the first and second chakras (lower belly). Place your hands on the lowest part of your belly and push your belly out with the in breath. Use the pressure of your hands on your belly to feel into the area. Breathe several times into this place. Then, begin to isolate your breath on your upper chest. Place your hands there, and again feel the rise and fall of the chest. Spend some time here.

When you are just beginning this exercise, practice moving your breath, isolating it to your belly for a while and then to your chest for a while. Continue to breath into these areas several times a day. This is a new skill, so be easy on yourself. Don't be judgmental if this is hard for you. Finding these new places in your body is a journey in and of itself. I have found that some people are naturally chest breathers while others are more belly breathers. Once you can connect the breath within the isolated areas, you have mastered phase one and can move to phase two.

Phase Two

After you have mastered phase one, add the midsection into the equation, isolating the breath within three areas: the chest, midsection, and the lower belly. In phase two, you will assess the chest, midsection, and belly to determine the easiest and the most challenging area of isolation. Start with the easiest area, work your way up to the hardest, and end the session with the easiest again. First, bring your hands to the area that moves with the most ease—the area of your body that naturally moves with each passing breath. Start here and focus on isolating the breath within this area only. Now, explore the area that you perceive to be the hardest or most "stuck." Bring your hands to this area for several breaths. Throughout the day, repeat this as many times as needed in order to bring you back to your internal peace. Return to this place of ease and grace whenever you need to make a decision in life.

Adding Affirmations

Once you have completed phase two, I encourage you to up the ante. Breath work and affirmations work very nicely together. Choose short affirmations to use in conjunction with your breath work, and state them aloud before each inhale. This is a beautiful way to incorporate both practices together. You may also want to consider playing soft and nurturing music. Whatever steers you in the direction of relaxation!

FIVE

Herpes FAQ and Facts about Pregnancy

*Life is not about waiting for the storms to pass. It's about learning how
to dance in the rain.*

—VIVIAN GREEN

The Truth Revealed: Questions and Answers

Over the years, I have fielded thousands of questions from women
with herpes through my private practice, e-mails, Web sites, phone
calls, personal conversations, support groups, and as the educational
coordinator of a nonprofit, the Colorado H Club (H for herpes). What
is most shocking is that the same questions seem to arise again and again,
regardless of a woman's age or level of education. I have been able to help
these women of various educational backgrounds become empowered
with accurate knowledge of the virus.

This section provides you with some of the most common questions I receive. It dispels the myths and helps you to avoid the detrimental consequences of not knowing some fundamental facts. After reading this section, you will be equipped with answers well beyond the basics.

Q: What is herpes?

A: Herpes is a virus that causes skin infections, which often produce painful, itchy blisters. This virus has been around for 140 million years,[6] infecting humans and animals alike. Over twenty-five centuries ago, Hippocrates, the father of medicine, coined the term "herpes" from the Greek "to creep." Aptly named, herpes has the ability to creep along any nerve and infect skin cells at more distant sites.

Q: How does herpes hide out in the body?

A: Herpes can hide out in the body for many years during an inactive state known as dormancy. During these times, its home can be found just outside of the spinal chord in an area called the dorsal root ganglion. This is the time in which people mistakenly think they no longer have herpes because they have no symptoms. Periods of stress or a weakened immunity can cause the virus to become active again, also known as reactivation. The virus then leaves its home base and travels along nerves to the surface of the skin. This change from an inactive to active state often triggers symptoms most commonly associated with herpes including but not limited to itching, tingling, redness, and pain. As the body heals, the virus retreats back down the nerves to its home base in the dorsal root ganglia until it is reactivated again. In the case of genital herpes, the virus lives in the sacral region and causes symptoms in the genital area it innervates.

---

6 Christopher Scipio, Making Peace with Herpes: A Holistic Guide to Overcoming the Stigma and Freeing Yourself from Outbreaks (Green Sun Press, 2006).

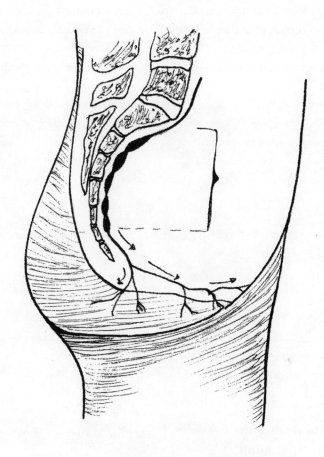

Side View of Pelvis and Sacral Nerve innervations

Q: Are there different strains of herpes?

A: Yes! Herpes has an entire family of viruses. Below is the list of the eight most common ones:

Herpes Simplex Virus HSV-1 and HSV-2: Oral and genital herpes. HSV-1 causes cold sores.

Varicella-Zoster: Also known as chickenpox or Herpes Zoster/ shingles.

Epstein-Barr Virus: Mononucleosis, also called mono or the "kissing disease," aptly coined for its transmission through saliva and kissing.

Ctyomegalovirus: Found in those who have weakened immune systems.

Human Herpes Virus 6: Roseola, a viral infection found in young children ages three months to four years. Symptoms include a high fever and small, slightly raised bumps.

Human Herpes Virus 7: Closely related to Human Herpes Virus 6, and poorly understood.

Human Herpes Virus 8: Kaposi's sarcoma. These lesions are classically found in AIDS patients.

Q: Does herpes simplex ONLY show up on the lips or genitals?

A: Herpes is a virus that can be found anywhere on the body. Anywhere there is skin or mucosal membranes, herpes can be found. People can become infected with herpes on their face, hands, legs, eyes, mouth, thighs, torso, or buttocks. Wrestlers are commonly infected with herpes gladiatorum on their bodies or herpetic whitlow on their hands.

Q: What is the difference between HSV-1 (Herpes Simplex 1) and HSV-2 (Herpes Simplex 2)?

A: In regards to symptom differences, genital herpes caused by HSV-1 tends to be a more mild form. It also tends to have a lower frequency of outbreaks. The genetic makeup between HSV-1 and HSV-2 is about 85 percent the same. Therefore, types 1 and 2 are essentially the same virus, when you consider the similarity of their DNA. HSV-1 prefers to live on the face, lips, and mouth. HSV-2, on the other hand, prefers to live below the waistline in what is called the boxer short region (the groin, genitalia, inner thigh, buttocks, and anus).

This location association is starting to change statistically, as we are seeing more and more genital herpes caused by HSV-1. The main reason for this is that more and more people are engaging in oral sex. Many people don't realize that a cold sore on the mouth can spread the herpes virus to the genital region, causing genital herpes. This route of transmission is on the rise in young people: amongst college age populations in the Midwest (US), the proportion of newly diagnosed HSV-1 genitally increased from 31 percent in 1993 to 78 percent in 2001.[7]

Q: How is herpes transmitted?

A: Herpes has three modes of transmission

1. Intimate Contact (horizontal transmission): usually kissing or sexual contact (oral or genital)
2. Autoinoculation: transmission from one area of the body to another
3. Congenital (vertical transmission): present at birth, passed from mother to newborn

Herpes is an infection that most commonly is spread by skin-to-skin contact, at a site where there is friction, a mucous membrane, or a break in the integrity of the skin. Herpes likes moist, warm, dark places and is killed pretty rapidly outside of the body. It is a parasite and as such needs a host to survive. During an outbreak, it is important to refrain from intimate contact. Proper hand washing with soap and water will kill the virus, so there is no need to obsess with hand washing every five minutes. As a precaution, it is also advised to properly clean any sex toys after use.

---

7 C. M. Roberts, J. R. Pfister, S. J. Spear, "Increasing Proportion of Herpes Simplex Virus Type I as a Cause of Genital Herpes Infection in College Students," Sex Trans Dis 30 (2003): 797–800.

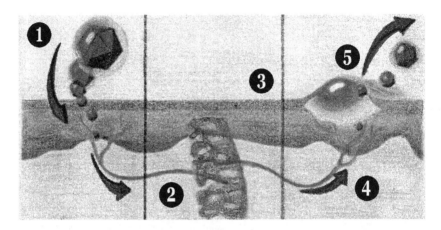

Transmission Of The Herpes Virus

Transmission of the Virus
1. The virus enters the body through the skin or mucous membranes.
2. After an initial infection, the virus settles in the nerves near the spine.
3. The virus enters a state of dormancy.
4. The virus is reactivated and travels along the nerve to the surface of the skin.
5. This reactivation causes another herpes outbreak: blisters, tingling, pain, and itching.

Q: Who gets herpes?

A: Anyone can get herpes. Herpes is so common globally that it has the second-largest incidence rate worldwide, trailing only behind the common cold.[8] Chances are you have been exposed to one of the herpes viruses at some point in your lifetime. Did you ever have chicken pox or mononucleosis? If so, you have been exposed to a member of the herpes family of viruses. Unfortunately, our society does not view the whole family of viruses equally. If you have herpes below the waistline, then you have genital herpes, an STD/STI.

According to the US Centers for Disease Control and Prevention (CDC), there are nineteen million new cases of STIs every year, which translates to about 52,054 people diagnosed daily. In March 2010, the CDC reported that one in six women and one in nine men have HSV-2. The University of California at Berkley showed that 60 to 90 percent of people carry HSV-1.[9]

I believe these to be very conservative statistics for a number of reasons. First, if studies have shown us that 85 percent of people who have HSV-2 don't know they have it, there are millions of people walking around who are not included in these statistics. Many who suspect they have herpes are often too embarrassed to get tested. I think that this mostly stems from our conservative roots in which sex and our sexual bodies are never to be discussed, even with our doctors. With more than fifty million people accounted for who have been diagnosed with HSV-2 in the US alone, it is time we talk about this taboo topic and get educated. Astoundingly, the diagnosis of herpes is on the rise despite the fact that most people never get tested.

Q: Do only the promiscuous get genital herpes?

A: Historically speaking, genital herpes was so common among prostitutes in eighteenth-century France that it was termed " a vocational disease of women"[10] But the answer to this emphatically is *no*: the promiscuous are

---

8 "NanoViricides Potential Herpes Simplex Virus Cure," NanoViricides, Inc. (August 10, 2009).

9 Michele Picozzi, Controlling Herpes Naturally: A Practical Guide to Treatment & Prevention, (Southpaw Press, 2006).

10 John Leo, "The New Scarlet Letter," Time (August 2, 1982).

not the only ones to get genital herpes! It is ridiculous that a virus that affects at least one in six women is still associated with promiscuity.

In the book *The Truth About Herpes*, a study was conducted in British Columbia, showing that "20 percent of women who have ever had sex have HSV-2. Once they have had six or more sexual partners, about 40 percent of women contract HSV-1 or 2, and after ten or more partners the risk on contracting the disease goes up to 60 percent."[11] I do not think these numbers reflect promiscuous behavior. In fact, there are many women who get infected with herpes after their very first intimate connection!

Q: What are the symptoms of herpes?

A: There are a number of symptoms that can occur with a herpes outbreak. The classic presentation follows a course of progression that often begins with a tingling feeling, also known as a prodrome,[12] followed by an irritation or redness on the skin (plate 1). Within a short period of time, tiny fluid-filled blisters appear at the site (plate 2). They are often painful and itchy. These blisters then begin to ooze, and the site becomes crusted over (plate 3). When the blisters burst, an ulcer or depression (plate 4) occurs, and a scab begins to form (plate 5). Generally, it takes two days to two weeks for the wound to heal.

---

11 Stephen L. Sacks, MD, The Truth about Herpes (Gordon Soules Book Publishers Ltd., 1997).

12 Fujie Xu, MD, PhD; Maya R. Sternberg, PhD; Benny J. Kottiri, PhD; Geraldine M. McQuillan, PhD; Francis K. Lee, PhD; Andre J. Nahmias, MD; Stuart M. Berman, MD, ScM; Lauri E. Markowitz, MD, "Trends in Herpes Simplex Virus Type 1 and Type 2 Seroprevalence in the United States," JAMA 296(8): 964–973, doi: 10.1001/jama.296.8.9642006.

The Phases of Healing

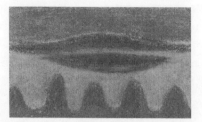

Plate 1

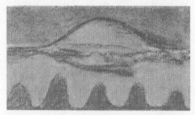

Plate 2

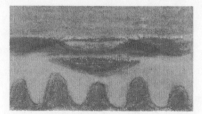

Plate 3

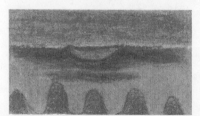

Plate 4

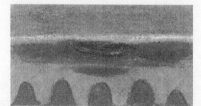

Plate 5

It is not uncommon for people to also have flu-like symptoms with an initial outbreak or subsequent outbreaks. I used to feel fatigued, my muscles would ache, and my lymph nodes would become swollen.

Q: Why do primary outbreaks or initial outbreaks usually create more intense symptoms?

A. For most people, the initial outbreak is the most intense because this is your body's first attempt to fight off the herpes virus. It can take some time to build up immunity, and as a result, subsequent outbreaks are generally less intense and often become less frequent. Some people are able to build up enough immunity that they can become symptom free. This does not mean that the herpes virus has left their body; rather, it has just gone into a state of dormancy.

Q: Can you have herpes and not have any symptoms? Not even a sore?

A: Yes. You can have herpes without *any* symptoms. One of the most challenging things about herpes diagnosis is that you might think you have a yeast infection, ingrown hair, jock itch, impetigo, or other skin irritations—but in fact you have herpes. This has made it very challenging for people to get properly diagnosed.

Although you could have only one or not any of these symptoms and still have herpes, some typical symptoms of genital herpes include the following:

- Blisters
- Sores
- Itchy areas
- Tingling areas
- Burning areas
- Painful urination
- Skin fissures and cracks
- Skin ulcers
- Swollen lymph nodes
- Fatigue
- Depression

- Pain down leg
- Flu-like symptoms
- Body aches
- Watery discharge from the penis or the vagina

Whether you've experienced symptoms of herpes or not, it is your ethical responsibility as a sexually active adult to get tested. Herpes is not part of a standard STI/STD screening, so if you haven't specifically asked to get tested for herpes, you probably have never been screened. Under all circumstances, if you get cold sores on your mouth, nose, or face, you have HSV1. While many deny this or are ill informed, a cold sore on the face is no different then a sore below the waist.

Q: Do the symptoms differ in women than men?

A: Research has shown that the symptoms in women can be statistically different than men. Below is a chart that outlines the difference between women and men during a primary or first HSV-2 infection.[13]

Symptom	Women	Men
Fever, malaise, headache	68%	39%
Pain at site of outbreak	99%	95%
Duration of pain	12 days	11 days
Vaginal or urethral discharge	85%	27%
Duration of discharge	13 days	6 days
Swollen lymph nodes	81%	80%
Painful urination	83%	44%

Q: Is there a difference between what men with herpes think they have and what women with herpes think they have?

A: Yes. The Virology Research team at the University of Washington compiled a list of symptoms that patients often confuse with herpes.[14]

---

13 L. Corey, "First-episode, Recurrent, and Asymptomatic Herpes Simplex Infections" (1, pt. 2), Journal of the American Academy of Dermatology 18 (1988): 169–72.

14 Charles Ebel and Anna Wald, MD, MPH, Managing Herpes: Living and Loving with HSV (American Health Association, Inc., 2007).

What Women With Herpes Think They Have	What Men With Herpes Think They Have
Yeast Infection	Folliculitis
Urinary Tract Infection	Jock Itch
Menstrual Complaints	Normal Itch
Hemorrhoids	Hemorrhoids
Heat Rash	Zipper Burn
Urethral Syndrome	Insect or Spider Bite
Allergy to condoms, spermacides, sperm, elastic/pantyhose	Allergies to condoms
Irritation from bike seat, shaving, douching	Irritation from bike seat, tight jeans, sexual intercourse

Q: Can you transmit herpes and not even know you have it?

A: One of the greatest paths of transmission is among people who carry the virus and don't know they do. If you are reading this book, you probably have symptoms of the herpes virus, and your viewpoint of the infection is colored by the physical reality of it. Current research is showing that this is in fact one of the many reasons why the transmission rates are so high. The largest study on genital herpes was conducted in 2006 by the National Health and Nutrition Examination Survey (NHANES). This survey included a type specific blood test done on several thousand people representing a cross-section of the US population.

It was discovered that only 15 percent of people who tested positive for HSV-2 reported any symptoms or history of genital herpes. That means that the other 85 percent of people who had genital herpes had no idea they had it! (See Figure 1.) Surprisingly, after the study educated the test population on the signs and symptoms of herpes, it was discovered that 70 percent of the people who tested positive where able to identify and recognize symptoms that had never been properly identified (Figure 2).[15] I have found this to be true more so with men than women and would ascertain that it is because women are more intimately cued in to their bodies and any changes that occur with them.

---

15 Xu et al, "Trends," 964–973.

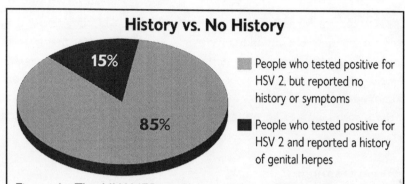

History vs. No History

15%

85%

People who tested positive for HSV 2, but reported no history or symptoms

People who tested positive for HSV 2 and reported a history of genital herpes

Figure 1 - The NHANES study showed that 85% of people with HSV 2 don't know they have it

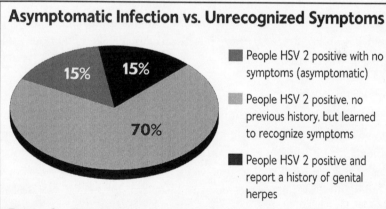

Asymptomatic Infection vs. Unrecognized Symptoms

15%   15%

70%

People HSV 2 positive with no symptoms (asymptomatic)

People HSV 2 positive, no previous history, but learned to recognize symptoms

People HSV 2 positive and report a history of genital herpes

Figure 2 - This figure illustrates the phenomenon of unrecognized herpes and the power of educating people about symptoms

Q: Does herpes cause cold sores?

A: Yes. Cold sores are caused by HSV-1, which is why they respond to over-the-counter creams like acyclovir, a herpes antiviral medication. Cold sores also respond to all natural ointments including red marine algae, lysine, aloe vera, beeswax, lemon balm, emu oil, and tea tree oil. Do not engage in oral sex if you have an active cold sore. This could result in the transmission of herpes to your partner and a subsequent genital herpes diagnosis to an uninfected partner.

Q: What is shingles?

A: Shingles is a painful rash most commonly appearing as a band or cluster on one side of the body. Shingles is most often found in adults with weakened immunity who had chicken pox as children. Much like the herpes simplex virus, the herpes zoster virus infects the nerve roots and therefore can lay dormant in the body for many years. Periods of stress, disease, weakened immune system, or medication can cause the virus to awaken from a dormant state. An active shingles infection cannot cause shingles in an uninfected person, but it can cause chicken pox to one who has never had it or had the chicken pox vaccine.

The prodrome of shingles can start with flu-like symptoms that later develop into a progression similar to HSV: itchy, tingling, red skin; fluid-filled blisters; ruptured blisters; ulcerations and/or scab. Some people do not get a full-blown rash, but for those that do, the healing process takes anywhere from two to four weeks. Medical treatment for shingles includes antivirals, antidepressants, and pain management. Several of the natural remedies listed in this book will also work for shingles. The good news is that most people do not get a reoccurrence.

Q: Has kissing ever been banned?

A: In ancient Rome, Emperor Tiberius banned kissing because it caused such a terrible epidemic of lip sores.[16]

---

16 Leo, "Scarlet Letter."

Q: What is autoinoculation?

A: Autoinoculation is the process in which the herpes virus infects a new area of the body in an already infected person. It is as if the person self-infects. An example of autoinoculation is if the virus jumps from above the waist to below the waist. This is most probably caused by improper hand washing after touching an open sore and then touching the genitals. Autoinoculation after the first outbreak is extremely rare. Generally, the body builds up enough immunity so that any future outbreaks have such low levels of virus (viral load) that transmitting it from place A to B on the body is nearly nonexistent. As a caveat, the virus *can* still travel along the same nerve route, and it would not be considered autoinoculation. Remember, the virus lives at the nerve root, so it can show up in any place along the path of the nerve as it travels to the surface of the skin. For example, if you have an outbreak in the genital region, it could move from the vagina to the anus.

Autoinoculation is more of a concern for children who frequently touch cold sores and then their nose or mouth. It is possible to transmit the virus to a new region if the skin is broken or you are touching a mucous membrane. Remember, the virus prefers moist, warm areas to live. It is important to have good hygiene, but you don't need to be obsessed. Unfortunately, I was one of the rare cases where it jumped ship from below the waist to above the waist. During that time in my life, I was very stressed out, and my immunity must have been compromised in order for this to happen. This is why I and every health-care professional will agree that the best defense for herpes is a strong immune system.

Q: Is it possible to get herpes in the eye?

A: Yes. This is called Herpes Simplex Keratitis or Ocular Herpes. It causes inflammation of the cornea of the eye, and its symptoms can mimic conjunctivitis. If you suspect that you have developed a herpes infection of the eye, it is paramount that you seek medical attention. This infection is the number-one cause of blindness in one eye in the US.

Q: Did my partner lie to me about his viral status?

A: I have fielded this question many times and the answer to it is not necessarily. Herpes mimics several other conditions, and as I have stated before, 85 percent of people who have herpes don't know it. Since herpes is not part of the standard STI panel, getting specifically tested for herpes is the only way to be certain of anyone's viral status.

Q: Will I always get an outbreak in the same place?

A: Generally, yes, but there are exceptions to the rule. It is possible for the virus to travel from the base to another "road" or branch in the vicinity of the initial outbreak. This is normally within inches of the initial outbreak. These main "roads" and branches are referred to as dermatomes[17] at the surface of the skin. Each band of gray represents a different nerve root. In general, the outbreaks tend to stay in the same banded area. Moving from one banded area to another is quite rare, and as a result, people tend to have reoccurrences in the exact location of the primary outbreak. Once the body has the opportunity to build up an immune response to the virus, other areas of the body become more protected.

---

17 Dermatome: an area of skin that is mainly supplied by a single spinal nerve.

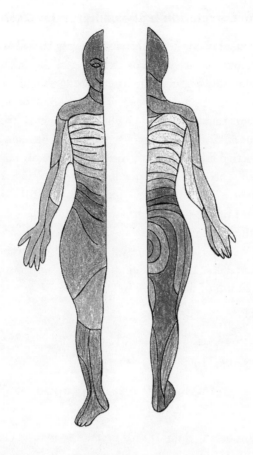

The Dermatomes

Q: Is HSV an STI or an STD?

A: HSV is an STD (Sexually Transmitted Disease) and an STI (Sexually Transmitted Infection). Some medical professionals are now referring to herpes as an STI (Sexually Transmitted Infection) instead of an STD. This name change is being made in an effort to decrease the stigma commonly associated with this chronic infection, which is so underreported and prevalent in our society. Since herpes is one of the most contagious STDs and it transcends all socioeconomic classes, races, and religions, it is not a virus of discrimination. Currently, the term STD is still being used interchangeably with STI in the medical community.

Q: What is the correlation between herpes and other STIs?

A: If you are sexually active, the chance of having an STI at some point in your journey is extremely high. For example, HPV[18] is common among 70 percent of the adult population, often causing genital warts or cervical dysplasia,[19] and a whopping 80 percent of the adult population has had chlamydia at some point in time.[20] One of the risks in having herpes is that it increases your risk for acquiring HIV and HPV. The main reason for this is that during active herpes lesions, the outer protective layer of the skin is compromised. This decreases your immunity to other STIs, making it easier for pathogens (virus, bacteria, fungus) to enter the body. If HIV or any other STI is present during intimacy and you have a genital sore that is not healed, there is a greater chance of acquiring the virus. If you are a sexually active woman, it is extremely important for you and your partner to get tested for STIs so that you can make informed decisions about your health and the health of those you love.

Q & A on Testing

Q: I am overwhelmed by the testing options. What is your advice?

A: The most important thing regarding testing is to make sure you are getting a type-specific test. A type-specific test is one that identifies whether or not you have type 1 (HSV-1) or type 2 (HSV-2) herpes.

Q: What is a swab?

A: A swab is a sample of cells, taken from a visible sore or a break in the skin where the herpes virus is thought to reside. Clinicians acquire a swab

---

18 HPV (human papillomavirus) is explained in great depth in the STD description and symptom chart.

19 Cervical dysplasia is also explained in the STD description and symptom chart.

20 Terri Warren, RN, NP, The Good News about the Bad News: Herpes: Everything You Need to Know (New Harbinger Publications, 2009).

by using something that resembles a Q-tip and vigorously rubbing it over a sore.

Q: Why would I get a sore swabbed when I could have a blood test instead?

A: If this is your first outbreak, a type-specific swab test will give you the fastest results.

Q: Is it too late to get a sore swabbed if it is already scabbed over?

A: No, but ideally the best time to get a sore swabbed is before it heals over. The greatest amount of virus is found in the blistered or open sore. As the body heals, over time the virus is slowly killed off and begins to retreat back to its home near the spine. As more and more virus is killed off, there is less and less of the virus to be swabbed, and the more likely you are to test negative for the HSV virus.

Q: How accurate is the culture swab test?

A: The culture swab test has a high rate of false negatives. This means that the test shows up negative when in fact you have the herpes virus. This is a common error with the test, and research has shown it occurs about 76 percent of the time.[21]

Q: What is a culture test?

A: A culture test is a sample, or swab, that is taken from your sore, and then combined with healthy animal cells to see if the herpes virus becomes active or present.

Q: What is the best blood-specific test?

A: The PCR or polymerase chain reaction test is the test I most frequently recommend for its accuracy and price point. PCR is a DNA-based test that can be used in swabbing and blood testing.

---

21 Ibid.

Q: How long does it take the virus to show up in a blood test?

A: Typically, it takes about three months from the time you are exposed to have enough antibodies for a blood test to show up positive.

Q: If I am having a PCR blood test done, why might my doctor want to do another swab test?

A: The PCR blood test can tell you what type of herpes virus you have but cannot tell you where that virus is. The swab test allows you to identify if you have HSV-1 or HSV-2 present at a specific sore.

Q: What is the western blot test?

A: This is the most accurate blood test available, which makes it the gold standard. Unfortunately, the test is also very expensive, technical, and it is only performed at the University of Washington. The western blot test is only recommended when test results are inconclusive.

Q: I think I have been infected with the herpes virus, but I have no sores. I know that I have to have a blood test done, but I don't want to wait three months to get tested. Can I get tested earlier?

A: Yes, you can get tested earlier, but know that the accuracy of the test will increase with time. The chart below reveals the accuracy rates in regards to the length of time passed after becoming infected.[22]

3 weeks after infection:	50% of those infected will test positive.
6 weeks after infection:	70% of those infected will test positive.
16 weeks after infection:	Almost everyone who is infected will test positive.

Q: How long do I need to wait to receive my tests?

A: In general, most clinics will get the results back within a week or so.

---

22 Terri Warren, RN, NP, The Good News about the Bad News: Herpes: Everything You Need to Know (New Harbinger Publications, 2009).

Q: Why isn't herpes included in a standard STD panel?

This is a great question, and depending on whom you ask, the answer could be different. I personally *do* think that it should be included in a standard panel. There are sexually responsible adults who get tested for STDs, receive a negative test result, and assume that they are free of *all* STDs, including herpes! Most people who are tested for STDs have no idea that they must specifically ask for a herpes test. This false sense of security gives people a license to go willy-nilly about their sexual lives! Not only are our clinicians giving their patients a false sense of security, they are also contributing to the massive unconscious transmission of the herpes infection. On the contrary, here are some arguments that support the decision to *not* include it in a standard panel.

- One argument is that adding herpes to a panel is an unnecessary additional cost, since herpes is so common anyway.
- A woman I spoke with from the CDC stated "off the record" that since herpes does not lead to any terminal disease or illness, it does not pose a risk to public health. This is the "it's just a rash" position.
- I spoke with the head of an STD clinic in the Pacific Northwest who stated that the fear among clinicians is that they might mis-diagnose an infection that has such a huge stigma attached to it. After challenging him on the accuracy of blood typing, he *still* felt that the approximately 3 percent error of misdiagnoses was way too much of a risk to expose someone to an emotionally charged, incurable, scarlet-letter diagnosis.
- Other clinicians believe that a positive test for herpes would not change a person's behavior.

Questions about Diagnosis

Q: Do doctors ever misdiagnose herpes?

A: Yes. It wasn't until the 1940s that herpes was found to be an actual virus. Then, 1960's research started to isolate the virus into two types that we know today: HSV-1 and HSV-2. Although it is said that the virus was misdiagnosed all the way through the 1970s, the truth is, it's *still* being misdiagnosed.

It used to be that doctors would diagnose herpes based on classic presentations of painful, itching blisters. This "classic presentation" is now debunked due to the alarming number of people who never elicit such classic symptoms. Type-specific blood testing, which enables us to differentiate between HSV-1 and HSV-2, was not available until more recent years. The older tests could only reveal a positive or negative result for the herpes virus. This was extremely limiting in regards to helping patients determine their level of risk and how they might have acquired the infection.

Doctors still misdiagnose herpes all the time. Herpes has been called the great masquerader because it can look like so many different things. We need to get doctors on board with proper diagnosis of herpes so that we as patients can be empowered, educated individuals.

Q: I get cold sores in the winter but now have a new rash on my genitals. Is it herpes?

A: If you get cold sores, then we already know that you have HSV-1 and it would show up in a blood test. What you don't know is whether or not this new rash is HSV-1, HSV-2, or something else. The only way to be sure is to have a type-specific test. If your sore is new, it is too early for HSV-2 to show up in your blood. Instead, get it swabbed and let your health-care provider know that if it is positive for herpes, you want to know if it is type 1 or 2. If the test comes back negative, you are not out of the woods yet. Sometimes swab tests are not able to detect the virus. Since it takes time for the virus to show up in your blood, get a type-specific blood test in three months to be certain that you don't have genital herpes.

Q: I had my sore swabbed and it came up negative. Could I still have herpes?

A: Yes. In order for a test to show up positive, there must be an adequate amount of virus in the sore. If the sore is nearly healed, or if it is a reoccurring sore, there might not be enough of the virus for the test to show up positive.

Q: I have cold sores, which I know is HSV-1. I just broke up with my partner who had HSV-2. Did I get the infection?

A: It's uncertain. You will need to get a type-specific blood test for HSV-2. Some are as easy as a finger prick with a ten-minute result period.

Q: I had a blood test done, and it was positive for HSV-1. Does this mean I have genital herpes?

A: Not necessarily. What it means is that you have antibodies to the HSV-1 virus. A blood test cannot tell you the location of the virus. Only an open sore can tell you the location of the virus. If it is on your lip, it is a cold sore; if it is below the waist, it is genital herpes.

Q: I have sores, and my doctor thinks it's herpes. She sent a swab test to the lab and it came back negative. A month later, I had the sores appear in the same spot. I went back to my doctor and she conducted another swab test. This time it came back positive. What should I believe?

A: There are many reasons why you initially tested negative for the herpes virus. When getting tested, it is important to do so within the first forty-eight hours of your first occurrence of the appearance of sores. If your sore is scabbed over or not in an active period, it will be harder for the swab to pick up the herpes virus. This would result in a negative result when in fact you do have herpes. When a test result comes back positive, you can pretty much bet on it. Test results that come back positive are incredibly accurate.

Q: Five months ago I presented to my doctor with sores in my genital area. My doctor sent out a swab test and it came back negative. I am now having a second occurrence in the exact same place. Should I have another swab test done?

A: Most likely your doctor will want to do a blood test. Since it has been more than three months from your initial symptoms or exposure, your body has had the opportunity to produce antibodies, which then can be detected in the PCR blood test. The doctor might also want to do another swab test.

Q: I am sexually active and have not had any symptoms for HSV-1 or HSV-2, but would like to get tested anyway to determine if it's present in my body. What should I do?

A: Because you do not have any symptoms for herpes, a blood test is your only option. Remember, it takes three months from the time you were exposed for the virus to show up in your body.

Q: Do doctors ever purposely lie about a herpes diagnosis?

A: Yes, this does happen. I now suspect that the doctor who initially diagnosed me with impetigo on my face was trying to "protect" me from the correct diagnosis of herpes simplex. Not only are patients being misinformed by blatantly keeping herpes outside of the traditional panels, they are being lied to when doctors might suspect herpes simplex. I was shocked when I read Terri Ward's book, *The Good News about the Bad News*. Here is an excerpt:

> Sometimes clinicians tell people who have suspicious rashes on their hips or buttocks that they have herpes zoster, even though the clinicians actually suspect or even know that their patients have herpes simplex. As time has passed and I've interacted with more and more clinicians around the country, I've discovered that this strategy is more common than I'd ever imagined. It isn't done maliciously and is intended to protect patients from what's believed to be "really bad news," and perhaps also to avoid "opening the can of worms" a herpes diagnosis requires. Some of those clinicians even consider my personal approach of correctly diagnosing as many HSV-2-infected people as possible to be intentionally harmful and insensitive to the feelings of perfectly nice people.

Q & A on Herpes and Partners

Q: How do I protect my partner if I have herpes?

A: Even if you do not have symptoms, you can still transmit the virus to your partner. According to a University of Washington study, "simply avoiding sexual contact during the active phases of infection provides enough protection for more than 95 percent of susceptible men and more than 81 percent of susceptible women per year."[23]

The best way to protect your partner is to abstain from sexual contact during any active symptoms and to use a protective barrier like a condom or oral dam. Unfortunately, a protective barrier is only as good as the area that it covers. For example, if you have herpes on the inner leg or groin, a condom would not cover the infected area. In addition, do not use spermicides, condoms, or diaphragm jelly that contains nonoxyldol-9 (N-9). This is an ingredient that irritates the vagina and cervix, causing lesions and increasing the risk of herpes and other STI transmission.

I also encourage women to always urinate after sexual intercourse. This allows for a cursory, natural cleanse of sorts and helps to decrease infection and irritation from pathogens. Since we never can be certain whether or not we are shedding the virus, there always poses some level of risk for a noninfected partner.

To help decrease the transmission of the virus to your partner, you should consider using a personal lubricant that contains carrageenan.[24] Carrageenan is a naturally occurring polysaccharide extracted from red seaweed that has been shown to be effective in decreasing the transmission of several viruses. Since carrageenan is a naturally occurring substance, it can never be patented. Fortunately, this will help to keep the cost down. This substance is currently being used in personal lubricants like Divine 9 and as a protective barrier on condoms. There have been studies done in mice that suggest that carrageenan is a powerful microbicide that can kill the HSV virus upon contact. This natural ingredient works by attaching itself to the outside of the HSV virus, preventing it from infecting new cells.[25]

Even though no studies have been done in humans, I suggest using an edible personal lubricant that contains carrageenan. In addition to using

---

23 Sacks, Truth.

24 C. B. Buck, C. D. Thompson, J. N. Roberts, M. Müller, D. R. Lowy, et al, "Carrageenan Is a Potent Inhibitor of Papillomavirus Infection," PLoS Pathog 2(7) (2006): e69, doi: 10.1371/journal.ppat.0020069; M. J. Carlucci, L. A. Scolaro, M. D. Noseda, A. S. Cerezo, and E. B. Damonte, "Protective Effect of a Natural Carrageenan on Genital Herpes Simplex Virus Infection in Mice," Antiviral Research Nov. 64(2) (2004):137–41.

25 Vanaja R. Zacharopoulos and David M. Phillips, "Vaginal Formulations of Carrageenan Protect Mice from Herpes Simplex Virus Infection," Clinical and Diagnostic Laboratory Immunology, July 1997, p. 465–468 1071-412X/97.

a condom, apply this lubricant in and around the genital area to further prevent transmission.

A quick summary:

1. Know the facts about transmission.
2. Abstain from sexual contact if you have any symptoms of an outbreak.
3. Use protective barriers such as condoms and dental dams.
4. Do not use protective barriers or sexual-enhancement gels containing nonoxyldol-9 (N-9).
5. Urinate after sexual intercourse.
6. Use a personal lubricant containing carrageenan.
7. Encourage your partner to lead a healthy lifestyle. If you are infected and your partner is not, it is important that you both keep your immunity high. This can reduce transmission rates.

Q: How often do I shed the virus?

A: It is possible to transmit the virus even when you don't have any symptoms. This is known as asymptomatic shedding, which means the virus is active at the surface of the skin, but you might not experience the normal prodrome or outbreak. The current research shows that the virus sheds an average of 4 to 13 percent of days of any given year.[26] This means that in any given month, the virus will shed an average of one to four days. Unfortunately, much more research needs to be done on viral shedding. There can be vast differences in the results, depending on how frequent the data is collected and how accurate the measurements are. I have seen these statistics as high as 60 percent and as low as 1 percent. It is possible to decrease the asymptomatic shedding with prescription drugs, but as with any prescription drug, this too poses a health risk.[27] In addition, some viral strains have become resistant to the use of current therapies.[28] When in doubt, abstain or use a condom or dental dam.

---

26 Ebel et al, Managing Herpes.

27 Ibid.

28 Warren, Good News.

Q: Is it possible in a long-term relationship to never transmit the virus?

A: Here is the good news: there has been research conducted that shows some long-term couples never transmit the virus to one another. Dr. Charles Prober from Stanford studied such common discordant[29] couples in which one partner had HSV-2 and never transmitted it to his or her long-term partner.[30] It was discovered that the more encounters the couple had with one another without transmitting the virus, the less likely it was to occur. In general, however, after several years passed, an event occurred that broke the barrier to infection, and transmission would occur. This was usually due to a mistake, a choice, or asymptomatic shedding.

Over time, many couples outweighed the risks and chose to live their lives as if the virus were no big deal. We evaluate risks every day, whether it is in driving a car, flying a plane, going rock climbing, or even crossing the street. Risks exist in many of our daily activities, but the power of choice backed with accurate information is what is important here.

Q: My doctor suggests that my partner be placed on an antiviral as a preventative measure. What is your opinion?

A: I once consulted a couple in which the woman was positive for HSV-2 and the man was negative for both HSV-1 and -2. The woman was so fearful of transmitting the virus to her new love that she did everything in her power to be responsible. The man loved her so much that he said herpes was not a deal breaker at all. At her request, the man took an antiviral medication, Valtrex, every day as a prophylactic. This shocked me! This was the first time I had spoken to a couple in which the noninfected partner was taking an antiviral. I felt that this was risky. Since the current drugs on the market act by stalling the synthesis of viral DNA, they interfere with natural reproduction of the virus and can cause drug-related toxicity. I encouraged the man to be proactive in naturally building up his immunity in order to defend the virus, as opposed to taking a drug that probably decreased his overall immunity and that produced only speculative results at best.

---

29 Discordant indicates one person in the relationship has herpes while the other person does not.

30 Sacks, Truth.

I think the there are three main things to learn from this couple. Firstly, herpes gifts us with the opportunity to review our health and to make healthy choices. Secondly, it gives us the chance to encourage our partners to take hold of their health and to build up their defense system. Finally, when love strikes, herpes often becomes a topic of "how do we manage it" versus "will it destroy us."

Q: If my partner and I have the same type of herpes, can we pass it back and forth to one another?

A: This is a common question, and the answer is no. If two people have the same type, then they already have the antibodies to defend themselves. It is, however, possible to be infected with one type and still be at risk for being infected by the other. This is one of many reasons why it is very important to get tested, so that you can determine your level of risk when becoming intimate. If you do have type 1, it partially protects you and makes it harder for you to get type 2.

Q: If I don't have symptoms, can I still transmit the virus to my partner?

A: Yes. There is always a risk of asymptomatic shedding. This is when you don't have symptoms, but you still could transmit the virus.

Q: Are women more at risk than men?

A: Yes, consider our anatomy. Herpes is not a conversation that impacts only women, but according to Dr. Stephen Sacks, women are statistically three to four times more at risk than men,[31] and an alarming 48% percent of African American women are reported to be carriers.[32] According to Dr. Kevin Leone, 50 to 70 percent of unmarried women in the US ages forty-five to fifty have genital herpes HSV-2.[33] Although the overall number of confirmed carriers of genital herpes has increased over the years, there

---

31 Ibid.

32 F Xu, MD, PhD, MR Sternberg, PhD, SL Gottlieb, MD, SM Berman, MD, LE Markowitz, MD, et al., "Seroprevalence of Herpes Simplex Virus Type 2 Among Persons Aged 14-49 Years-United States, 2005-2008," Morbidity and Mortality Weekly Report (MMWR), April 23, p. 456-459 59(15)/2010.

33 Accessed on NPR.

still exists an enormous amount of undiagnosed carriers. If more people were correctly diagnosed and educated about herpes, it would not carry such stigma and fear.

Q: My partner's STD test was negative. Could he/she still have herpes?

A: Yes. A standard STD test does not screen for herpes, so unless your partner has been tested specifically for herpes, you will not know whether or not he/she is a carrier.

Here is our story...

When I first asked Richard, my husband, if he had ever been tested, he said that every year he went to get a routine physical, which included an STI panel, and that he was as healthy as a horse and had "stellar" lab results. Among other things, he had low blood pressure, low cholesterol, high HDL, and no STIs. As his old-school Dr. Welby doctor sat across from him in his cute bow tie, he declared that Richard was one of his healthiest patients. Now why would Richard think otherwise? He held me in a loving embrace and basically said that he loved me no matter what and wanted to pursue our relationship. My intuition told me that he was the man I would marry, so I never insisted that he get tested. We were both off the market and were willing to take the risk of transmission.

A couple of years later, Richard was working on launching a new business and was very stressed out. He noticed that there was "something" on his penis, and he asked me to check it out. I did and was shocked that it appeared to be herpes. Now, here is a man who knows as much about herpes as anyone would, in living with a doctor who specializes in it. He was all on board for me creating a platform for other women to learn more about herpes and to reclaim their physical and emotional vitality. I asked him a handful of questions, and after about five minutes, he remembered the first time he'd had something like this. It was in college, several years ago when he lived in Hawaii. He even remembered the girl that he was with! He assumed, like many men, that it was just some kind of irritation or an ingrown hair. It itched a bit, but he did not think much of it.

It would be very easy for us to assume that he had acquired the virus from me, but after questioning him we both realized that this rarely recurring skin condition was most probably from his college years. We both realized that this rare, recurring skin condition was most probably herpes. We still to this day do not know if it is herpes because the results from the test would not change how we live our lives. He still does not think it is herpes, and I am quite certain that it is. We will probably have him do a blood test at some time, just to eliminate the uncertainty, but at this point it is of no priority. It is just a skin condition that comes up every few years for him, and he barely thinks about it. He is fortunate in that he doesn't live his current life any differently, but it does make him question whether or not he ever exposed anyone else to it.

Since you have read this far, I can reveal my one exception to everyone needing to get tested. If the results would in no way alter your sexual practices in a monogamous relationship in which both parties are knowledgeable about all of the risks, then there is no need to get tested.

Q: I think I have herpes symptoms; could it be another STD or an STI?

A: It is possible. Below is a list of the most common STDs, their symptoms, and some alternative treatment options.

STD: HPV

Human papilloma virus is mostly associated with abnormal Pap smears and cervical dysplasia. It is also a virus that has a life cycle that is virtually unpredictable. It can cause genital warts, an STD, and some forms have been linked to cervical cancer. There are many different strains of HPV, some of which are mild and will disappear and heal on their own accord. Some strains, if not detected, can cause cervical dysplasia. Cervical dysplasia describes abnormal cells in the area of the endocervical canal or cervix. Without intervention, these precancerous cells could develop into cervical cancer. The immune system plays a key role in the management of HPV, maintaining normal cell growth, and replication.

SYMPTOMS: Chronic inflammation of the cervix, chronic vulvar pain, and warts are all symptoms associated with HPV, although some women have no symptoms at all. This is why early detection with routine Pap smears is recommended.

DID YOU KNOW?

HPV is a mysterious virus. The HPV virus is linked to cervical cancer because the virus invades the already weakened cells within the cervical area. A depressed immune system creates the environment for the virus to thrive. Chronic physical and emotional stress greatly impacts the ability of the immune system to function properly.

There are scientific studies that show a direct correlation between the emotional health of a woman and the severity of her dysplasia. Women who are negative, passive and pessimistic in emotionally stressful situations are more apt to have difficulty flushing these abnormal cells from their body. They also experience more severe symptoms than those who are more positive emotionally. It has been found that women who have more mild dysplasia cells often have better coping skills when dealing with stressful situations. These women were more optimistic and actively sought out solutions to their problems. Since the cervix is associated with the second chakra, sufferers of HPV should investigate any negative energy associated with sex, money, creativity, or relationships. This negativity could be impeding the healing process.

TREATMENT: Antioxidants can help heal and prevent cervical dysplasia. Vitamins C, A, and E, folic acid, and beta-carotene have been proven to be very beneficial.

STD: Gonorrhea

Gonorrhea is a curable infection that is caused by a specific bacteria, *Neisseria gonorrhoeae*. The growing concern about gonorrhea is the increase in resistance to antibiotics. It is usually transmitted through anal or vaginal sex, while also being transmitted via oral sex. It can affect the rectum and/ or joints, but usually causes inflammation of the genital mucous membranes.

SYMPTOMS: While men usually show symptoms, women do not. It is not uncommon for women to be misdiagnosed with a vaginal or bladder infection, when in fact it is gonorrhea. Those who do develop symptoms will do so within ten days of being infected. Symptoms include cloudy or bloody discharge from the vagina, burning during urination, frequent urination, and pain during intercourse. If not treated promptly, PID (pelvic inflammatory disease) and fertility complications can occur.

STD: Syphilis

Syphilis is a sexually transmitted disease associated with the microorganism, *Treponema pallidum*. This microorganism can cause painless lesions, also called chancres, within any organ or tissue, but most often occur on the mouth, genitals, or rectum. It is a disease that can lie dormant in the body for decades, but when active, can severely damage many organs including the heart and brain. This STD is often found in men with HIV.

SYMPTOMS: There are four stages.

1. Primary Syphilis- Within three weeks of becoming infected, a painless sore, or chancre, appears. This occurs at the initial site of contact.
2. Secondary Syphilis- About 6-8 weeks after an initial infection, a rash may appear, spreading all over the body and can include the palms of the hands and the soles of the feet. This "great imitator" disease can also produce fever, sore throat, muscle aches, loss of appetite and many other symptoms associated with other common diseases. These symptoms may come and go throughout the year.
3. Latent Syphilis- This is the stage of dormancy where there are no symptoms.
4. Tertiary Syphilis- In this late stage, the disease becomes dangerous, possibly developing complications in the brain, nerves, eyes, heart, blood, liver, joints, and bones. This can occur a year after the initial infection or several decades later.

DID YOU KNOW?

While holistic drugs and methods are used to treat many STDs, it is highly stressed that syphilis only be treated by pharmaceutical drugs. It is a serious, debilitating, and potentially life-threatening illness, and its recommended treatment is penicillin. Homeopathic medicine has proven to be beneficial in conjunction with other medicines in order to prevent long-term consequences.

STD: Chlamydia

Chlamydia is a group of microorganisms that cause inflammation of the regional lymph nodes and lesions on the genitals. It can infect the cervix, throat, eyes, and urethra. More commonly, it infects the fallopian tubes, uterus, and upper genital tract. It is the most common STD within the United States, and the number of people infected continues to grow.

SYMPTOMS: While this disease is often symptom free, it is a very dangerous disease as it can cause pelvic inflammatory disease, which can be life threatening. Mild symptoms of pain during sex, painful urination, abdominal pain, and vaginal discharge can be present.

DID YOU KNOW?

Natural approaches aimed at improving immunity are key here and should only be used in conjunction with conventional treatment. After a course of antibiotics, it is important to repopulate the gut with probiotics.

STD: Pubic Lice (Crabs)

Pubic lice are tiny insects found in your pubic area, resembling little sea crabs, visible to the human eye. They lay eggs and feed on blood, causing very itchy bites.

SYMPTOMS: If you see tiny insects in your genital areas, including thighs and abdomen, or have severe itching, are all sure signs that you have pubic lice.

STD: HIV

Human immunodeficiency virus can cause a life-threatening condition, AIDS. HIV interferes with the body's ability to fight disease-causing organisms. It can be spread through infected blood, breast-feeding, pregnancy, and sex. There is no cure. Medications and lifestyle changes can be implemented in order to prolong life.

SYMPTOMS: Fever, headache, rash, and swollen lymph glands are all symptoms within the first couple of years, although some do go symptom free. As the virus continues to gain strength, mild and chronic infections and conditions begin to develop: weight loss, diarrhea, swollen lymph nodes (often the first sign of HIV), cough, shortness of breath, and fever.

DID YOU KNOW?

Those who implement raw and organic foods into their diet seem to improve immensely. Enemas help to rid the system of toxins and cleanse the colon, where the disease is harbored. Increasing supplemental intake of vitamins A, E, B, and C are often encouraged. Acupuncture has been known to help decrease symptoms as well. This is a disease that is successfully managed by several alternative medical approaches.

STD: Genital Warts

HPV is the organism that causes this skin disease.

SYMPTOMS: Warts can be flat, undetected by the human eye, or raised, which can be singular and small or more cauliflower-like in appearance. They are moist and soft and can appear red, pink, white, or dark in color. The area of infection may burn or itch.

> Note: If you have genital warts, please educate yourself more on HPV and cervical dysplasia, as they are all heavily intertwined.

DID YOU KNOW?

Many genital warts resolve on their own without ever causing any health problems. Sexually active individuals will most likely be infected with warts at some point in their life without ever knowing it.

An ointment composed of vitamin A and the herbs Thuja and Lomatium has been used as a holistic ointment to treat genital warts. This is one of many alternative solutions for healing genital warts. Also, white vinegar will often visually "light up" warts, although this is not diagnostic.

STD: Trichomoniasis (Trich)

This rather unknown single-cell parasite causes vaginitis within some infected women.

SYMPTOMS: An odorous discharge, as well as itching and redness of the infected area are all symptoms. Greenish-yellow vaginal discharge, odor, pain, itching, or light vaginal bleeding can all be symptoms.

DID YOU KNOW?

If you have vaginitis caused by trichomoniasis, a diet low in fats, sugars, yeast, and refined foods is highly recommended. Many who have vaginitis also have an overgrowth of candidiasis or yeast. Candida flourishes in a diet high in sugars. Adding probiotics and garlic to your diet can greatly improve the symptoms of vaginitis.

Herpes and Pregnancy: What Are the True Risks to the Newborn?

What is it about herpes and pregnancy that places us all in fear? The mere thought of exposing our newborns to a disease that could range in severity from a tiny skin rash to their death can be debilitating and can lead us to believe that the dream of delivering a normal, healthy baby is no longer an option. My initial diagnosis of herpes did not lead me to ponder the potential death of an unborn child, for I knew that those statistics were incredibly rare, but I did imagine what it would feel like passing a stigmatizing disease on to my otherwise perfect newborn.

Before I got pregnant, I wasn't thinking much about my herpes outbreaks. I had learned how to manage my herpes symptoms and knew that the chance of having a baby with neonatal herpes was extremely low. Statistics were in my favor, and the numbers were reassuring.

Neonatal herpes—herpes of the newborn—is not even considered a reportable disease, according to the Centers for Disease Control and Prevention (CDC, a branch of our public health system whose sole purpose is to monitor diseases worldwide). If the CDC does not list neonatal herpes as a reportable disease, then I think it's fair to say that you don't need to be overly concerned about the potential of a newborn dying from your genital herpes. However, neonatal herpes is something you need to be educated about so you can decrease the likelihood of transmission. Here are some facts that I hope you will find comforting:

- Neonatal herpes is extremely rare. A three-year study in Canada (2000–2003) revealed a neonatal HSV (herpes simplex virus) incidence of 5.9 per 100,000 live births (.00006 percent) and a case fatality rate of 15.5 percent.[34]
- Herpes during pregnancy is common. Upward of 25 percent of all pregnant women have herpes. Have you ever heard of a woman whose baby had herpes? I highly doubt that you have! Does this help to put your risk into perspective?
- Eighty to ninety percent of neonatal herpes cases are from women who didn't know they had it. Therefore, women who know they have herpes can greatly reduce the risk of transmission. Sharing your herpes status with your health-care provider will greatly reduce transmission.
- Most neonatal herpes is managed effectively with treatment.
- The most common neonatal symptoms are rashes. These rashes are easily managed and treated.

It is my intention to equip you with the facts so that fear of transmission doesn't consume you during your pregnancy. Remember that even though genital herpes is quite common, neonatal herpes is uncommon. The majority of neonatal herpes cases are manageable, mild skin rashes that are not fatal. For example, a herpes rash on a baby's scalp is not fatal, nor is it sexually transmitted. This sort of skin rash is not much different than a cold sore, which is also caused by the herpes virus. At some point in your child's life, he or she will likely encounter the herpes virus! Herpes is a virus that includes many common strains you might be familiar with including chicken pox or mononucleosis; HSV-1, which causes cold sores; or shingles, Epstein Bar, and roseola.

---

34 Kropp RY, Wong T, Cormier L, Ringrose A, Burton S, Embree JE, Steben M, et al., "Neonatal Herpes Simplex Virus Infections in Canada: Results of a 3-year National Prospective Study." Pediatrics, June 2006, p.1955-62 117(6).

Take these facts to heart and allow them to diminish your fear of the unknown and mysterious "what if" scenarios running rampant in your mind. Remember that the likelihood of your child being exposed to herpes from someone other than yourself is as high, if not higher, than being exposed by you. Aunts, uncles, grandparents, and friends get fever blisters, right? These loved ones are just as likely to expose your infant.

The Power of Antibodies

If you are reading this book, perhaps you have been diagnosed with genital herpes and are thinking about getting pregnant. The odds are stacked in your favor. Women who go into pregnancy with genital herpes pass on herpes antibodies to their unborn child. This is good news because it is these antibodies that become a part of your baby's developing immune system. In other words, if your baby is exposed to herpes, your antibodies will help kill off the virus. Nature has already equipped us with an arsenal to fight off unknown pathogens like herpes. Your maternal antibodies will also help to protect your baby against E. coli, staph, and many other potential pathogens. If you breast-feed your child, you will continue to pass on these antibodies and help your child to build his or her developing immune system. Breast-feeding helps build immunity and provides your child with essential nutrients that cannot be substituted with any supplement. The fact is:

> Ninety-eight percent of all newborns are exposed
> to viruses and pathogens and are born healthy.

Why some babies succumb to illness while others do not is something of a mystery. The exposure to herpes and the development of neonatal herpes is no different. When weighing out the facts, don't forget that herpes is not the only thing your infant is exposed to. He or she is also exposed to all sorts of bacteria, viruses, and fungi. It's just part of the human experience. You cannot shield your baby from the world of pathogens. Chances are, his or her immune system will engage, and your baby will be just fine.

Q: If I have herpes, what should I tell my OB/GYN or my health-care provider?

A: If you are pregnant and know that you have genital herpes, inform your health-care provider of your herpes status. You should know exactly what strain of the virus you have. Is it herpes type 1 (HSV-1) or herpes type 2 (HSV-2)? If you don't know, request a type-specific test. You will also need to know the STD status of your partner. If you both have herpes but your partner has a different strain than you do, you are at risk for contracting the other strain. You need to know the specifics to decrease the risks of transmission to your unborn child. During labor and delivery:

- **Do not allow fetal monitoring,** because it has been identified as a risk factor for transmission. It is thought that the electrodes placed on an infant's scalp can create tiny breaks in the skin, thereby opening a route of transmission for the herpes virus.
- **Do not allow for the premature rupture of membranes.** It is not uncommon in the hospital setting for a doctor to prematurely rupture the membranes in an effort to speed up the birthing process. The longer your membranes stay intact, the more protected your baby will be. This premature break in the membranes can also increase the risk of contaminating the birth canal.

Q: If I have herpes, can I still have a vaginal delivery?

A: Yes, yes, and yes! Having genital herpes does not keep you from having a vaginal delivery, but if you are experiencing an active outbreak during labor, your doctor will probably suggest a Caesarean. Every outbreak is unique, and the decision to deliver naturally should be discussed with your health-care professional.

It's important that you talk to your health-care provider about your herpes status so he or she can best manage your pregnancy. Take the time during your pregnancy to nurture yourself. Eat well, take naps, meditate, and take time to celebrate your pregnancy.

Q: Does genital herpes affect my ability to get pregnant?

A: No, genital herpes does not affect fertility. This is true for both women and men.

Q: If I do not have genital herpes, but my partner does, what should I do during pregnancy?

A: First of all, I would get a blood test done to see if you carry the antibodies for either HSV-1 or HSV-2. You might think that you don't have herpes when in fact you might. If it is determined that you do not have herpes 1 or 2, then it's imperative that you protect yourself during your pregnancy. Herpes acquired during pregnancy accounts for nearly 80 percent of the neonatal herpes cases.

During pregnancy, if you and your partner have different strains of the virus, I recommend that you abstain from intercourse and oral sex. This is most important during the third trimester. If, however, you discover that you both have the same strain of the herpes virus, then you should be safe to have unprotected sex during times when neither party has symptoms.

Q: If I do not have herpes (I've been tested), but my partner does, what should I do during my pregnancy to prevent neonatal herpes?

A:

- Refrain from intimacy when your partner is having any symptoms of a herpes outbreak, including but not limited to itching, tingling, blisters, and redness.
- **Do not** have intercourse during your third trimester, *period*. This is when you have the greatest risk of transmission to your newborn.
- **Do not** have oral sex if your partner has any lesions or symptoms in his or her mouth.

Q: Can I breast-feed my baby if I have herpes?

A: Absolutely! I am a huge advocate of breast-feeding. If by chance you get a herpes outbreak on your breast or nipple, simply pump and discard the milk from the affected breast and continue nursing with the unaffected breast. If both breasts have sores or symptoms, pump and discard the milk until all lesions have healed. This will allow your body to continue to produce milk. In the meantime, supplement your milk with baby formula.

Q: Are cold sores contagious to my newborn?

A: Yes. If you or a loved one has an outbreak on the face, do not kiss the baby or allow him or her to touch your sore. If your child does touch your sore, simply wash his or her hands with soap and water. During nursing, you might want to consider a mask if your infant is prone to touch your sore.

Q: If I have active lesions during labor, what's the likely course of action?

A: If you are having an active outbreak during labor, your physician might recommend a Caesarean, depending on where you live. In the United States, according to the American Medical Association, the standard of care has been determined that a Caesarean is recommended if lesions are present in the boxer shorts region. This, however, does not totally eliminate the risks of transmission. If you are in the UK during labor with a recurrent outbreak, your doctor will not routinely offer a Caesarean section.[35] The NICE (National Institute of Clinical Excellence) in England recently concluded that pregnant women with a recurrent HSV should be warned of the uncertainty of the effect of planning a Caesarean to reduce the risk of neonatal herpes. They do not believe at this time that there's sufficient data to warrant a Caesarean to reduce the transmission of neonatal herpes. As a result, it's important that you talk to your health-care provider about your herpes status to see what options you might have, while constructively evaluating the risks involved. For example, a sore near or in the birth canal poses more of a threat than a sore on your inner thigh.

Q: If I am having an outbreak and my water breaks before my scheduled C-section, what should I do?

A: Contact your doctor immediately. When your membranes rupture, this creates a wet path for the virus to travel from a sore outside your body to inside your body. A C-section will probably be immediately called for.

---

35 National Collaborating Centre for Women's and Children's Health, et al., "Caesarian Section- Full Guideline Draft.", September 2011, p. 17.

Q: If I am prone to frequent outbreaks, what can I do to increase my chances of a vaginal delivery?

A: Decreasing the overall stress in your life, eating well, exercising, and supplementing with vitamins and minerals are paramount in helping build up your immunity.

It is not uncommon for women who have recurrent outbreaks to have an increase in outbreaks during their final trimester. Some doctors would also recommend the use of the antiviral acyclovir as a preventative after week thirty-six of your pregnancy. Personally, I would only use this course of action if I were having frequent outbreaks throughout my pregnancy. Since acyclovir's mechanism of action is at the genetic level, I would not feel comfortable exposing my unborn child to this. On the other hand, I believe that increasing your chances of a vaginal delivery outweigh this potential risk if you are exhibiting frequent outbreaks.

Q: If I have frequent outbreaks, am I more at risk for transmitting the virus to my unborn child than someone who rarely has outbreaks?

A: No. It has been determined that the risks are the same. I would, however, encourage a woman who is having frequent outbreaks to seek out care. In most cases, outbreaks can easily be managed naturally.

Q: If I have genital herpes, will my doctor have to continually give me tests and visual inspections?

A: Absolutely not! I can tell you from personal experience that my midwife did not have to do an internal exam until sometime in my third trimester. If you are having symptoms, it is important to communicate this to your provider.

Q: If I have genital herpes, am I still a candidate for a home birth?

A: Yes! I can honestly tell you that our choice to use a midwife and to have a home birth was one of the best decisions I have ever made. I felt so supported and cared for in my journey of pregnancy and birth. Our midwife provided us with amazing pre- and postnatal care. She treated me like a queen, answered all of our questions, and properly managed my care when things arose. Birthing our daughter, Madeline, in the privacy of our own home was the most magical moment of my life. A midwife will be able to offer you the best of care!

Q: I get cold sores on my lips. Do I need to take any drugs during pregnancy to decrease the chances of transmitting it to my unborn child?

A: No, you do not need to be on any antivirals during pregnancy. It is important, however, that you do not kiss your baby when you are having an outbreak on your lips. Once your sore is healed, you can kiss your baby as much as you would like. It is also important that you not let any family or friends kiss your baby when they have a cold sore on their lips.

Q: I have genital herpes and have been on daily suppressive therapy. Should I take my antiviral medicine during my pregnancy?

A: Medical guidelines would suggest stopping your antiviral until week thirty-six of your pregnancy; however, you need to discuss your options with your attending physician. There has not been enough research to discover the safety of using antivirals throughout the entire pregnancy. I am an advocate of bringing your focus to building up your immunity naturally, because the best defense to herpes is a strong immune system.

Q: Why is it that acquiring herpes during pregnancy is associated with greater risk?

A: Surprisingly, only 2 percent of the population acquires herpes during their pregnancy, and it is this group who is at the highest risk for transmission, especially during their third trimester. These are the reasons behind this: the first outbreak...

1. is usually the most severe
2. has the highest viral load in the sores
3. often includes lesions on the cervix
4. has not given your body the opportunity to build up antibodies that can then be passed on to your unborn child

Q: Why don't doctors traditionally test for herpes during pregnancy?

A: I still find it mind-blowing that even though herpes is one of the most common STDs, doctors do not screen for it during pregnancy. It is still not recommended by the governing board of obstetrics and gynecology to administer a herpes test as part of the standard STD panel. I believe that this decision is based on the fact that the risk of neonatal herpes is quite low. If 85 percent of people who have herpes don't know it, then a lot of normal babies are being born from mothers that unknowingly have herpes.

Q. I have genital herpes, and my baby has a rash. Could it be herpes?

A. A herpes rash on an infant looks similar to a herpes rash or outbreak in an adult. Neonatal herpes rashes can take a few weeks to develop. The rash most likely will be found on the point of presentation during a vaginal delivery. If the baby was delivered head first, the rash might be on the head; foot first might show up on the foot, buttocks first might show up on the buttocks. The rash will start out as red; then it will form a cluster of tiny blisters that will rupture, ooze, ulcerate, and heal—just like the progression in an adult.

If your baby has a rash, don't automatically assume it's herpes. The good news is that rashes in healthy newborns are quite common. Neonatal herpes rashes can be easily confused with other rashes like milia, a common infant rash that appears as tiny white dots and will heal on its own. The more serious forms of herpes, although extremely rare, have either no symptoms or common ones such as irritability and high fever. If you are concerned about your infant, seek out professional counsel.

Q: If my baby or older child does get a herpes rash, how should I treat it?

A. You can treat it topically as you would with an adult. Be mindful that if your child will touch the area, you will want to cover it with a bandage. You may use aloe vera, colloidal silver, an antiviral herpes balm, or an essential oil like Melissa or lemon balm diluted in vegetable oil. Internally, check with your pediatrician before implementing any remedies.

SIX

Hidden Triggers and Toxicities

When health is absent wisdom cannot reveal itself,
art cannot become manifest, strength cannot be exerted,
wealth is useless, and reason is powerless.

—HEROPHILOS, 300 B.C.

The Toxic Umbrella: Heavy Metal and Chemical Toxicity

What do heavy metal and chemical toxicity have to do with herpes? *Everything!* The more toxicity you have in your body, the weaker your immunity and the more frequent your outbreaks will be. Our modern world has exposed all of us to several toxicities. This environment has lead to an increase in many chronic diseases including heart disease, asthma, type 2 diabetes, autism, and cancer. It is not a matter of if you have heavy metal toxicity; it is more of a matter of how much you have.

Industrialization, with its smoke stacks and waste products, has polluted the air we breathe, the water we drink, and the food we eat.

If you were grown in the belly of your mamma, you are toxic! Toxicity is passed from mother to child. There was a study done in 2005 by the Environmental Working Group to determine the level of toxicity in the umbilical chords of ten newborns. According to the report, called "Body Burden—The Pollution in Newborns," here is what they discovered:

- 287 chemicals identified
- 180 chemicals identified as known carcinogens
- 217 cause brain toxicity
- 208 cause birth defects or abnormal development in animals[36]

It goes to show you that the process of being born puts you at risk for toxic exposure. This is why you *must* cleanse your body and refuel it with nutrients. Not only are our bodies' mineral profiles out of balance because of the nutrient-deficient foods we eat, but essential minerals are being replaced by toxic ones. When the body does not have an essential mineral it needs, it will use an element that most closely resembles it. For example, mercury and zinc have similar enough properties that if the body does not have enough zinc, it will try to use the neurotoxin[37] mercury instead. When zinc is replaced by mercury, our body cannot run properly, and it becomes a toxic dumping ground. Since minerals are like spark plugs, eventually your body gives out and succumbs to disease.

Toxic Food and Why We Need to Supplement

The best way to assess your exposure to heavy metals and your basic mineral profiles is through hair mineral testing. After analyzing several hair mineral analysis lab results and studying under the tutelage of Dr. Lawrence Wilson, MD, I have learned a great deal about nutrition, vitamins, minerals, heavy metal toxicity, and detoxification. What has shocked me most is that everyone I have ever tested has shown both toxicity and mineral imbalances. The root of our problems stems from the

36 July 15, 2005.

37 A neurotoxin is an element that is toxic to the nervous system.

environment we live in, the stress in our lives, the food we eat, the air we breathe, and the thoughts we think.

Even in the 1930s, our government recognized the depletion of our soils and the overall decrease of nutrients in our food. Modern agricultural practices and processed foods have only added to our widespread mineral deficiencies. Since plants receive their minerals from the soil, years and years of soil depletion have left our produce weaker than it once was. Our farmers are not replenishing the soil with the minerals that have been stripped over the years. For example, you would probably have to eat eight bowls of spinach today to absorb the nutrients in one bowl of spinach your grandparents ate. So, not only are our fresh foods "weaker," but conventional farming also riddles them with genetic modifications, pesticides, and other harmful substances. The bottom line is that we need to be eating more organic fruits and vegetables, period!

Fruits and vegetables have so many vitamins, minerals, and phyto-nutrients (plant nutrients) that it is vital that we consume more of them. When you look at your plate of food, you should ideally see lots of color. With our Standard American Diet being as SAD as it is, it is of utmost importance that we supplement our diet with vitamins and minerals. Even if you have a pristine diet of organic fruits, veggies, nuts, and meats, you still need to supplement because of soil depletion. These depletions wreak havoc on our body over the long run, resulting in several chronic diseases. Herpes is no different in that if you don't clean up your diet and restore the vitamins and minerals that your immune system needs, you will be constantly riddled with outbreaks. The body must have the proper building blocks to run a tight ship.

That being said, most people are malnourished and toxic. This is why it is important to clean up your diet and determine your degree of toxicity. I have found Analytic Research Labs to be the best company to assess your level of toxicity through their hair analysis service. Unfortunately, not all companies that do hair analysis are equal. Some wash the hair before they analyze it, which produces inaccurate results. Hair tests enable us to determine what your body has been doing for the past few months, what toxicities exist in your body, what minerals are out of balance, how your immunity is functioning, and many other systemic evaluations. This valuable information allows a practitioner to create a unique supplement program for each individual.

The program that is outlined in this book includes general supplement guidelines that will help your body to detoxify naturally and rebalance, whether you decide to have a hair test or not. This supplement program will flood your body with nutrients and allow it to begin the detoxification process. In doing so, your body will naturally begin to remove toxic chemicals and heavy metals from your system. This is chelation therapy by addition, not subtraction, because your body will naturally release heavy metals as it utilizes more preferable minerals in your diet and supplement regimen. Unfortunately, quick fixes like detox foot baths and IV chelation therapy[38] are successful in removing heavy metals, but they also deplete us of all of the other minerals in the body. This is because these quick fixes act as large magnets, pulling out the heavy metals in the body, while also extracting the healthy minerals in our body, all of which are also ionically charged. There are foods and supplements, like kelp, that offer a superior mechanism of natural chelation. Kelp is one of my favorite natural chelators because not only does it pull out heavy metals from the body, but it also helps to nourish and rebalance the thyroid with healthy iodine. I have found that most Americans have unhealthy thyroids, and the need to support this gland is so important to our health.

A Common Mineral Imbalance

One of the most common mineral imbalances that I have witnessed in hair tests is the deficiency of zinc and the toxicity of copper. As with all minerals, we reference them as a married pair of sorts because they have such a great synergistic relationship. There are known ratios of these mineral patterns that are ideal for health. One of the most important mineral pairs to discuss for a person suffering from herpes is the copper/zinc balance. A copper/zinc imbalance has an enormous impact on immunity, hormonal function and the gorgeous, sexy skin we all strive for. As a result, this imbalance can frequently trigger more herpes outbreaks. In addition, the toxic load of heavy metals such as lead, aluminum, mercury, arsenic,

---

38 In IV chelation therapy, EDTH is used to draw out heavy metals, essentially working as a heavy metal magnet. IV chelation therapy is often used for patients who suffer from atherosclerosis (plaque in the arteries).

cadmium, and several other heavy metals could also be distressing your immune system and your body's ability to keep herpes dormant.

The good news is that a copper toxic/zinc deficient person must follow many of the same protocols as a person with herpes. If you do have this imbalance, it is of even greater importance to avoid seeds (except flax and hemp), nuts, and chocolate. These foods are high in copper *and* high in arginine, a double whammy for people with herpes because both could potentially trigger outbreaks. When people with herpes begin to supplement with fifty milligrams of zinc per day, they often get great results. The zinc helps to counteract some copper toxicity *and* it also helps you to rebuild your immunity. As a side benefit, zinc supplementation is a secret for great skin, and what does herpes affect? Your skin!

While I encourage you to eat more veggies (you can never have too many), I do *not* recommend going vegetarian. A vegetarian diet sets you up for this copper/zinc imbalance. Vegetarians in particular need to supplement with zinc because the phytic acid found in plant foods interferes with the absorption of zinc. In addition, although zinc is found in vegetables, it is in much higher concentrations in animal products. When we do not consume animal products, we are more at risk for developing zinc deficiency and copper toxicity.

Cosmetics and Personal Care

As women, we are always attempting to look our best. Historically, cosmetics have helped us to do this. I have never been one to wear lots of makeup, but over the years I have learned more about the handful of products that I use. One of the best things someone once told me is this: if you can't eat the ingredients of a product, it probably shouldn't be on your skin. Now, I can't say that I have gone to this extreme, but as a doctor I know that the skin absorbs a great deal of what we place on it. This is why some drugs are given as creams. The cosmetic industry has used harmful chemicals in their products for years, some with the intention of us having to rely on their products for the very reason we use them. For example, many body lotions contain alcohols that are toxic drying agents. At first these lotions appear to moisturize, but over time they dry us out. Did you know that several ingredients in our self-care products are derived from petroleum? How about the fact that some mascara is made from bat poop? I won't go into a litany of how one chemical company's toxin becomes a cosmetic company's binder or filler. The EU has banned many of the toxins we find in our food and cosmetics. Long story short, cosmetics are filled with ingredients that lead to cancer, birth defects, infertility, and organ damage. Do your research on a product before using a product on your skin, and go all-natural whenever possible.

WARNING: For those of you who get outbreaks on your face, I would not recommend the use of antiaging mechanical exfoliator devices that vibrate back and forth on the skin, nor would I recommend using any harsh exfoliators. These devices and products tend to agitate the skin and can cause outbreaks.

Top 10 Cosmetic Toxins
Mercury
Lead acetate
Formaldehyde
Toluene
Petroleum distillates
Ethylacrylate
Coal tar
Dibutyl phthalate
Potassium dichromate
2-Bromo-2-Nitropropane-1, 3 Diol

The Pits!

Most deodorants on the market are high in aluminum, which is very toxic to your body. High aluminum in the body has been linked to breast cancer, Alzheimer's, and dementia. Even the "all natural" salt deodorants contain natural aluminum, which is toxic. The only thing that I have found that is all natural, aluminum free, and effective is the deodorant made by the company Dermalogica.

Do you know the difference between a deodorant and an antiperspirant? A deodorant masks the odor whereas an antiperspirant is designed to block your glands from perspiring. Never use an antiperspirant! If you can't sweat, you can't eliminate toxins, and they begin to build up in your system. This is the precursory to disease.

Tampons

Did you know that tampons contain harmful chemicals like bleach and synthetic fibers? Unless you are buying all-natural tampons, your risk to such exposure is extremely high. Now think about where you are placing these products! Our skin and especially our mucous membranes easily absorb chemicals they come into contact with. Avoid generic, toxic tampons at all costs…especially if you suffer from genital herpes or HPV. You do not need to be adding any detoxifying challenges to your already depressed immune systems. If your body is a temple and you truly embrace your sexuality and goddess nature, then you *must* be mindful of the substances your expose your body to.

Electromagnetic Pollution

Have you ever thought about how electromagnetic radiation might be stressing out your body and contributing to your outbreaks? Stress leads to disease, and EMFs (electromagnetic frequencies) produce stress on our bodies. As humans, our bodies have the ability to adapt to new stresses, but unfortunately, it takes time to do so. The advent of cell phones, computers, cell phone towers, microwaves, and video games has come at a great cost, the overall impact of which might take time to see. Several studies are showing how EMFs contribute to fatigue, dizziness, loss of concentration, and tumors. If we could actually see how these devices pollute our environment, we might begin to think differently about them. Check out www.antennasearch.com. Based on your zip code, you can identify how many antennas are within your local area.

Why is this important? Our bodies work off electrical impulses and signals. Take, for example, the heart. In order for it to beat, it must receive an electrical impulse to do so. What happens when you bring two microphones close to one another? Interference! This is no different than our bodies coming into contact with these EMFs. Imagine how they might be affecting the impulses in your brain and heart!

We are seeing the rates of cancer skyrocket, which basically means that our immune systems are in overwhelm. I have a young businessman friend who was diagnosed with terminal brain cancer, and I seriously wonder how technology might have contributed to it. Dr. Andrew Weil, MD, author of *Spontaneous Healing*, states, "EMF may be the most significant form of pollution human activity has produced in this century, all the more dangerous because it is invisible and insensible."

How to Reduce Your Exposure to Electromagnetic Pollution

Use your cell phone on speaker or get an ear bud. This will increase the distance between your brain and the emitting signal, which will decrease the intensity of the signal zapping your brain. Check out the ear buds available on Dr. Mercola's Web site at www.DrMercola.com. I highly recommend subscribing to his healthy newsletter.

Don't use a Bluetooth either. This emits a signal, too, which could be harmful to your health.

- Consider purchasing a BioPro chip or other device that helps to protect you from EMFs.
- Turn your electronic devices off at night to give your body a break. This will also allow your computer to run more efficiently.
- Place your EMF hot spots, like your Internet hub, farthest from your bed and your children's beds
- Do not place your laptop on your lap to work (EMFs close to your reproductive area is not a good idea).
- Take your cell phone out of your pocket (they emit signals even while you are not using them).
- Limit "wired in" time for yourself and your children. Turn off the TV, Wii, and computer and read a book or play an interactive game like Cranium. Engage the mind, laugh, and connect to the ones you love. This will enhance your life instead of sucking it dry of mindless and often negative programming and media. As a side note, keep cell phones away from young children. Their sensitive brains are still developing!

There's Something Fishy Going On

Hidden metal and chemical toxicity is found in highest concentrations in large fish like tuna (don't forget that tuna fish salad comes from tuna), mahimahi, and swordfish. Our oceans have become a dumping ground, and the small fish live and feed themselves from this toxic soup. The big fish then eat the small fish. The concentrations of mercury and other toxins increase as the fish get larger and larger. Therefore, the bigger the fish, the greater the toxicity.

When we eat the fish, our body has a challenging time eliminating the toxins. The end result is that these heavy metals get lodged in our bones, brains, kidneys, and liver, wherever the body can "hide them," wreaking havoc on our immunity. *The Cove*, a documentary about dolphins, explains how heavy metal toxicity from eating fish is causing neurological disorders in some Japanese children. Eliminate the seafood that has the highest amounts of mercury from your diet, and substitute with seafood containing lower amounts of mercury.

Seafood Highest in Mercury

King mackerel	Shark	Swordfish
Marlin	Tilefish	Tuna
Orange roughy	Bigeye	Ahi

Seafood Lowest in Mercury

Anchovies
Butterfish
Catfish
Clam
Crab (domestic)
Crawfish/crayfish
Croaker
Flounder
Haddock
Hake
Herring
Mackerel (N. Atlantic)
Mullet
Oysters
Perch (ocean)
Plaice

Salmon (canned, fresh)
Sardines
Scallops
Shad (American)
Shrimp
Sole
Squid (calamari)
Tilapia
Trout (freshwater)
Whitefish
Whiting

Identifying and Removing Toxins from Your Life

(🌍) Be aware of the seven food products banned in Europe still available in the US:

- GMOs (genetically modified organisms)
- Stevia
- Bovine growth hormone
- Chlorinated chicken
- Food contact chemicals
- Herbicides, fungicides, and insecticides
- Food dyes

Feeling overwhelmed by all of the toxins in your life? Start with a mindful makeover of your home. Here are the areas to focus on removing toxic ingredients. Once you remove these ingredients from your home, you will be less likely to purchase them again. Replace toxic cleaning supplies with "green" ones, which will be better for your health *and* better for our environment.

The refrigerator and freezer
The pantry
The bathroom
Under the sink

Here are some specific tips to help you get started. If this is all [new to] you, take it one step at a time. Implementing change gradually will [have] the most lasting impact.

- Do your best to choose with fresh produce and meat: nonorganic foods contain veterinary drugs, pesticides, and heavy metals.
- Dispose of aluminum and copper cookware: these metals leach into our food.
- Buy fluoride-free toothpaste: fluoride is toxic and displaces healthy calcium and other minerals in your body.
- Remove mercury and other metal amalgams from your mouth: seek out a holistic dentist because your fillings could be emitting toxic metals each day, bit by bit.
- Drink spring water: it has less toxins and healthy minerals.
- Reduce consumption of canned foods: The aluminum from the cans leaches into the soil, and the liners often have phthalates and other toxins.
- Use only aluminum-free deodorant: aluminum leaches through the skin and has been linked to breast cancer and Alzheimer's.
- Go green with your cleaning supplies: your skin is the biggest organism, and an average cleaning product on the market contains heavy amounts of toxins like bleach, which then absorb through your skin and nose into your body. There are naturally occurring disinfectants you can use instead. Go to your local store and buy a natural or clean brand-name supplies, or opt to construct your own. Some products I recommend are Mrs. Meyers, Seventh Generation, Method, and Earth Friendly.
- Go all natural with skin, hair, and cosmetics products: toxins found in these products are carcinogenic (cancer causing) and cause birth defects, infertility, developmental abnormalities, and organ damage.
- Store food and water in glass: plastic containers and aluminum foil leach toxins.
- Avoid seafood with highest levels of heavy metals.
- Get a filter for your shower: remove chlorine and other toxic products for the water in your shower.

ations: this is a strong statement, I know, but the
[..]ve done has led me to the belief that vaccines do
[..]han good. Not only are they filled with toxins like
[...]merisol, and foreign DNA, they are also linked to
[...] disorders, ADHD, and other nervous-system disor-
[...]do your homework before vaccinating yourself or
[...]!

- Replace table salt with sea salt: table salt is heat blasted, chemically treated, and damaging to our body. Sea salt, on the other
hand, is alive and contains naturally occurring iodine and many
healthy minerals and micronutrients in proportions that are better for our bodies.
- Do your best to eliminate high-fructose corn syrup and foods that
are highly processed from your diet. If you can't read the label,
put it back. Fresh is best!

I most recently had a woman who joined our Pink Tent community
and attended a Women's Brunch. She sheepishly walked in the door and
worried that the dish she brought to pass was not organic. She shared her
"confession" with me and I assured her that all was well and that I don't
even eat 100% organic. I do my best, but it is very difficult to be organic
all the time. I watched as she took a deep breath and unwrapped her dish
to share. Never underestimate the power of infusing food with love, joy,
gratitude and prayer.

A Solution to the Toxic Umbrella

Our Standard American Diet (SAD) is filled with toxins that slow down
our bodies' ability to heal. These toxins include medications, heavy
metals, pesticides, alcohol, food preservatives, marijuana, drugs, and
several other foreign materials. Over time, our large and small intestines
get backed up and accumulate a thick layer of plaque from these toxins,
including undigested food and sometimes parasites. If you do not have a
bowel movement after every meal, then you have accumulated years of
junk in the gut. This thick layer of garbage decreases your body's ability

to absorb nutrients and maintain health. The only way to "refurbish" your gut is to do a cleanse that can scrub away the debris and clear out the junk.

A healthy gut is composed of many bacteria, which aid in the digestion of food. When we take antibiotics, we kill off this normal flora or bugs of the gut. When this happens, the balance of the gut gets thrown off, and an overgrowth of organisms like yeast can begin to take hold. Yeast, the organism that causes candida, can lead to all sorts of problems, from vaginal yeast infections to sugar cravings (yeast feeds off of sugar). After doing a cleanse or taking a course of antibiotics, it is important to take daily probiotics, a blend of good bugs to repopulate your colon. Probiotics are found in yogurt, kefir, kombucha tea, and kim chi, or you can opt to supplement with a probiotic capsule. The higher the organism count and the more variety of culture strains, the better. Beware not to ever choose a probiotic food that contains high-fructose corn syrup! Read your labels.

A cleanse gives your body a break from caffeine, sweets, alcohol, processed foods, and meat. This alone is challenging for many people. A cleanse also gives your body the chance to take a break from digesting solid food and instead focus on removing toxins and extracting nutrients. It is important to know that not all cleanses are created equal. In my opinion, it is best to do a cleanse that floods the body with nutrients, like an organic juice fast filled with leafy greens, ginger, garlic, carrots, beets, and other veggies. Each vegetable or herb used can help to pull the toxins out of your body. I don't recommend using too many fruit juices because they tend to spike blood sugar too much, which places a strain on the pancreas. Unfortunately, a water fast like the "Master Cleanse" has become very popular, but in my opinion it releases toxins in the body too fast and can leave you very depleted.

If you are new to cleansing, I recommend doing the colon cleanse offered by Life Force International. If, however, you already have a few cleanses under your belt, I recommend doing the colon cleanse from Blessed Herbs. I have found the Blessed Herb cleanse to go the deepest, which for some might be too much. The more toxic you are, the more likely you are to experience some cleansing reactions like headaches, diarrhea, rashes, gas, and abdominal pain. It is not uncommon to experience some of these symptoms while your body is releasing toxins. The Life Force cleanse is milder and easier to fit into a thirty-day gentle cleanse.

You might consider a colonic or enema if your symptoms become uncomfortable or you are not having at least a bowel movement a day.

If you do decide to do a cleanse, I recommend doing it during the spring and fall seasons. This is an ideal time because temperatures are milder and your body will better sync with Mother Nature's cleansing seasons. Harsh temperatures found in the summer and winter put an added stress on your body when you are attempting to heal. This added stress depresses immunity and makes it more challenging for your body to optimize energy for healing and removing toxins. Do *not* do a cleanse if you are pregnant or nursing.

My husband and I faithfully do our cleanses and consider them to be a cornerstone to our vibrant health. I have had patients report weight loss, allergy reductions, increased energy, improved immunity, improvement in digestion, and several other exciting changes. See the resource section at the end of the book for suggested cleanses.

The Top Ten Hidden Herpes Triggers Your Doctor Never Told You

Everything impacts your outbreaks: diet, exercise, supplements, immunity, stress levels, toxicities, environment—even your thoughts and emotions. Most doctors don't warn you about triggers that could be contributing to your outbreaks, leaving you feeling helpless and confused.

As a woman who has lived, loved, and thrived with herpes for fourteen years, I hope that in sharing my personal journey with you, we can move toward understanding and healing together.

Where I live in Boulder, Colorado, the high-altitude sunshine and heavy winds would often trigger my facial outbreaks in the winter, while sun and surf would trigger them in the summer. Pure bliss, feelings of ecstasy, hot yoga, hot tubs, saunas, and the dancing molecules of love were my main triggers. And two things in my life that brought so much joy to me, skiing and hot yoga, were both contributing to my outbreaks.

It took me some time to realize what my unique triggers were, but education is the gateway to empowerment. Know that as you heal, your body will become less and less triggered. Once you are aware of the potential triggers, you can make some changes and eventually determine your unique triggers. It's time to get empowered and learn how these simple changes and warnings can lead you in the direction of living a life free of outbreaks.

For some, herpes outbreaks act similarly to the red light on your car's instrument panel that lights up when the engine is overheating. Symptoms then become a signal that your body is overwhelmed and that it's time to make some changes. The good news is that there are changes you can make in your life to elicit healing, both physical and emotional. Here are the top ten triggers your doctor never told you about.

1. You're too stressed out. Stress is the number-one contributing factor to chronic disease. Stress depresses your immunity and therefore impacts your ability to keep herpes at bay. Managing your stress is one of the number-one things you can do for yourself *and* your overall health and well-being.

2. Your diet is high in arginine. Foods and beverages high in this amino acid are known to trigger herpes. Some foods high in arginine include nuts, seeds, coffee, alcohol and chocolate. Increase your intake of foods high in lysine including vegetables, chicken and eggs to counterbalance the arginine. If you are prone to joint pain or inflammation, omit nightshade vegetables from your diet.

3. You're dehydrated. A body cannot function properly when it is dehydrated. In keeping yourself well-hydrated, caffeinated and sugary drinks don't count! You need to be drinking at least eight glasses of clean water a day. If not, fatigue, tight muscles, decreased brain function and immunity, and increased pain, inflammation, and toxicity set in. Dehydration will slow down your healing process.

4. You're too hot! Too much friction and heat are triggers, be it in bed, at the spa, or at the gym. Consider the friction and heat generated by biking, running, vigorous sex, hot yoga, saunas, hot tubs, bathing nude, and sunshine (if your outbreak area is exposed to the sun). Beware.

Tip: if you suffer from genital herpes, don't hang out in your wet, sweaty tights too long after exercising. Herpes likes wet environments, too. Get chub rub when running? Use talc powder or a natural oil to decrease friction.

5. You're exercising too much or too intensely. This can be just as stressful on the body as not enough exercise. It can cause the adrenal glands to go into overdrive, producing a stressful state in which the herpes virus thrives. Consider taking at least one day off a week from your exercise regimen. Choose to do more gentle, nourishing workouts like yin yoga, swimming, or tai chi until you get your outbreaks under control.

6. You have a hormonal imbalance. A stressed-out and over-whelmed hormonal system can trigger outbreaks. This might be true if your herpes outbreaks occur at the same time every month. If so, considering finding an alternative health-care professional to balance out your hormones.

7. Your body is toxic. Your colon, liver, kidneys, and skin all work to process toxins. Did you know that the skin, aka the integumentary system, is the largest organ in the body? If it's struggling to eliminate toxins, then it will be challenged to keep herpes dormant. Some hidden toxicities might be found in your water, cosmetics, tampons, food, supplements, cleaning supplies, or environment. Toxins depress your immunity and impair your body's ability to heal herpes. This is especially true if you have never done a cleanse or you're constipated (not having at least one bowel movement a day). If you are constipated, you're reabsorbing your toxins. Is it time for you to do a cleanse and clean up your SAD (Standard American Diet)? Get your greens on!

8. You have a zinc imbalance. Zinc is paramount for proper skin health, immunity, and digestive health. White spots on your nails or indigestion could indicate a zinc deficiency.

9. Your sex life is "arginized." Condoms, spermicides, jellies, and sexual-enhancement gels often contain a secret herpes trigger: arginine. Be sure your sexy time is free of arginine.

Tip: Consider using a personal lubricant with the active ingredient carrageenan. This has been known to decrease the spread of STDs.

10. You have trauma in the pelvis. I have found that emotional and physical trauma in the pelvic area can trigger genital outbreaks. This trauma can be physical, like a car accident or surgery, or it can be emotional, e.g., sexual abuse. If the trauma is physical, I suggest chiropractic or craniosacral work. If the trauma is sexual, I recommend seeking somatic (body-based) therapy. Meditations, yoga, and chakra rebalancing are also quite supportive.

It is my hope that you're now able to clearly identify some potential triggers that you had never considered before. Start journaling the cycles of your symptoms, emotions, and lifestyle or dietary changes. This self-discovery will be indispensible on your journey toward wellness. Your healing path was uniquely designed for you!

Food: Know Your Peas and Carrots

> Let food be thy medicine and medicine be thy food.
>
> — HIPPOCRATES

Most Americans are clueless when it comes to a healthy diet. They are easily influenced by the latest, greatest fads on the market. Most people change up their diets in order to loose weight, but health is so much more than a target weight. As women, we rack up hours comparing ourselves to the skinny pinups on the front of every glossy magazine and media platform out there. There is no way we can compete with these women, who make up about 1 percent of our population. Sadly, many runway models are anorexic and heavily into drugs to maintain their Barbie-doll figures. This is not health, and in no way should you hope to be the airbrushed models in your minds. This will put you on the fast boat to depression, and in the meantime instead of getting healthier, you will be getting sicker.

Always remember that fad diets are often hard to follow long term and will leave you worse off than when you started. Eating should be about putting the proper nutrients and building blocks into your body so you can experience optimal health. As a culture, we are overweight and malnourished. Obesity is a huge health risk that we face as a culture, and if you fall into this category, it is paramount for you to make these changes *now*! Carrying around extra weight wreaks havoc on your health, and it greatly impacts your quality of life and leaves you much more at risk for chronic disease like heart disease, diabetes, arthritis, allergies, auto-immune disorders, gastrointestinal disorders, cancer...The list goes on. If you are not already taking prescription medications and you continue to follow the Standard American Diet (SAD), you will be left with the standard American health challenges.

The management of herpes is greatly influenced by the foods you eat. Whole, fresh, organic foods full of color and flavor are always best for the mind, body, and soul. Eat local, seasonal, and organic whenever possible to have the freshest of foods, to support your local farmers, and to decrease your carbon footprint. Food can be a medicine in and of itself, and the social aspects of eating well can be a blast. Sharing a plate of colorful, delicious, home-cooked food is *sexy*! The kitchen is a place where you can play and experiment with new flavors and textures. Stir up some love in your next meal; it nourishes the spirit, builds your emotional connection to others, and truly heals the body from the inside out. So slow down, break bread, and be merry!

At any given meal, most of your plate should be filled with veggies. What I love about vegetables is that they are filled with vitamins, minerals, and nutrients found in plants called phytonutrients. My favorite veggie powerhouses are kale, spinach, Brussels sprouts, carrots, beets, broccoli, and cauliflower. Think dark green, cruciferous, and colorful root vegetables. Veggies are low in sugar, high in fiber, and have many healing properties. Don't worry as much about going organic with the Clean Fifteen, the lowest in pesticides explained below.

When you are initially learning to manage your herpes outbreaks, I suggest you cut out the fruits in your diet and focus on green leafy veggies, beets, parsnips, carrots, avocados, onions, and garlic. Most people already have too much sugar in their diet, and although fruits have several nutrients, they are high in sugar. High sugar in the diet leads to weight gain, predisposes us to diabetes, and depresses our immunity. We need to keep our immunity strong if we want to put that herpes infection to sleep! A great idea is to weigh out a pound of vegetables each morning and commit to eating it by the end of the day. Take it on as a challenge, and be playful around it.

The key here is to get you in the habit of eating more vegetables. To start, you can eat these veggies raw, but ideally you want to cook most of them because it will be easier on your system to digest. For some people, it is easiest to blend the veggies in the morning as a shake. This is a great way to increase the vegetables in your diet, but it is as important if not more so to eat your vegetables cooked. The heat will begin to break down the vegetables so that it is easier for your body to extract the nutrients. If it is hard for you to increase the veggies in your diet, you must take a vegetable supplement. Avoid powders and pills with spirulina and chlorella due to their high prevalence of heavy metals.

The Dirty Dozen and the Clean Fifteen

The Environmental Working Group (EWG) coined the term "the Dirty Dozen" to identify the twelve fruits and vegetables that are known to have the highest amounts of pesticides. I suggest that when buying these foods you should do your best to go organic or be sure to wash them in water and vinegar. This will at least decrease your exposure to harmful pesticides. I keep a current list of the Dirty Dozen printed out by my grocery list. These are the most contaminated veggies and fruits in 2011. If you can't buy these organic, substitute with something else.

The Clean Fifteen, as you can imagine, fall exactly on the opposite side of the Dirty Dozen. While you can still aim to buy these organic, you can also buy them conventional. It's best to still shop locally if you can, or if anything, make sure you do a good job washing off the pesticides.

The Dirty Dozen

Celery	Peaches
Strawberries	Apples
Blueberries	Nectarines
Bell peppers	Spinach
Cherries	Kale/collard greens
Potatoes	Imported grapes

The Clean Fifteen

Onion	Pineapple
Corn	Avocado
Asparagus	Sweet peas
Mangos	Eggplant
Cantaloupe	Kiwi
Cabbage	Watermelon
Sweet potatoes	Grapefruit
Mushrooms	

Lysine and Arginine

One of the most universal recommendations specific to the management of herpes is to be mindful of the two amino acids arginine and lysine in your diet. Herpes outbreaks and many other chronic viruses are triggered by high amounts of arginine in the diet. Arginine feeds herpes and encourages its growth and reproduction. Lysine, on the other hand, boosts immunity and offers up protection from future outbreaks. Lysine is an antiviral that helps you heal naturally. So to sum it up, **lysine is our friend** and **arginine is our enemy**. Ideally, you want to decrease foods that are high in arginine and increase foods that are high in lysine. The higher the ratio of lysine/arginine, the greater its impact on keeping herpes dormant.

Although many people use lysine supplements, I do not recommend them as a daily protocol. Too much supplemental lysine will impair your immunity as much as too little lysine. Daily lysine supplementation also poses the risk of heavy metal toxicity. Food consumption is much more natural and totally safe. It has been shown that the effects of lysine supplementation are no better than the use of garlic, a much safer alternative.

Increase Foods High in Lysine

Most vegetables and fruits
Dairy-based products including cheese, milk, and yogurt
Fish, chicken, lamb, and beef
Brewer's yeast
Eggs
Avocado
Sprouts
Quinoa
Amaranth

Decrease Foods High In Arginine

All nuts and nut products
Nut butters (peanut butter, almond butter, etc.)
Caffeine
Chocolate
Seeds (except hemp and flax)
Oatmeal
Brown rice
Raisins
Whole wheat and white flour
Carob
Lentils
Wheat germ
Dried beans, including soybeans and tofu
Protein shakes, multivitamins, and body-building supplements that
    contain arginine

These latter foods should be eliminated from your diet until you are outbreak free for at least three months. At that time, you can slowly reintroduce them into your diet and see if they triggers any outbreaks. This process of elimination is the easiest way to learn more about your unique triggers. I have found that while some people are not triggered by high amounts of arginine, others are extremely sensitive. This is great information when you are learning about your triggers.

The above food recommendations are meant to point you toward managing your outbreaks and living a vibrant, healthy life. As discussed, there are many known triggers when it comes to herpes and certain foods. Over the years I have found people who are triggered to the point that even one bite of a high-risk food sends them right into an outbreak mode. I have also met other people who could pretty much consume everything on the list of triggers and not be affected in any way.

Frequent Outbreaks? Omit the Nightshades

If you suffer from herpes, not all vegetables are good for you. There is a class of vegetables called nightshades, which lead to inflammation and chronic muscle, joint, and nerve pain. During outbreaks, it is important to omit nightshade plants, the Solanacea family. Unfortunately, these vegetables tend to increase the inflammatory process, making symptoms worse. When you have herpes lesions, the skin is already irritated and inflamed. The last thing you want to do is fuel the burning fire from within. Are you feeling hot, hot, hot? If you are in outbreak mode or you are getting outbreaks frequently, I would avoid nightshade vegetables, fruits, and spices.

Nightshades are used in processed foods because they are addictive in nature. Maybe this is why I love Southwestern food so much! Some colas, like Dr. Pepper, have paprika or cayenne added to them. They are also hidden under the terms starch, natural flavors, and spices.

Nightshades to Avoid
- Veggies: tomatoes, peppers, eggplant, potatoes
- Berries: goji berries
- Tomato-based condiments: ketchup, hot sauce
- Processed foods: "starch," "natural flavoring," and "spices" in the ingredient list
- Spices: chili powder, curry, cayenne, paprika

Shopping Guidelines Summary

You are what you eat, from your head down to your feet! Not much has changed. If you can keep this in mind, simplicity is king. Here are the basics. If you don't know what the ingredients are listed on the label, stay away. But as always, label or no label, fresh is best! A healthy diet will improve your immunity and help your body keep herpes at bay.

When shopping for your food, do your best to use fresh ingredients and buy organic dairy, meat, and produce. If going 100 percent organic is cost prohibitive, start with organic meats since standard meat is chock-full of antibiotics, hormones, and other harmful substances.

Do most of your shopping on the perimeter of the store because the majority of the junk resides in the middle. If you can't pronounce or understand a specific ingredient on a packaged good, then it is probably not good for you. There are several hidden toxicities in packaged foods including high-fructose corn syrup, trans-fatty acids, monosodium glutamate MSG, and several other harmful preservatives.

- Don't use fad diets to reach your target weight.
- Add more color to your plate. More greens!
- Eat local, organic and fresh wherever possible.
- Limit your intake of fruits.
- Eat more cooked veggies.
- Avoid the Dirty Dozen and big fish.
- Increase the lysine and decrease the arginine in your diet.
- Consider decreasing or omitting the nightshades.
- Read labels.

SEVEN

Solutions: Self-Care Plan, Supplements, and Healing Remedies

A journey of a thousand miles begins with a single step.

—LAO TZU

Learning how to live, love, and thrive with herpes is a journey that starts with a single step in the right direction. Knowing where to start can feel overwhelming. The program outlined in this chapter incorporates lifestyle changes including dietary recommendations, supplements, and physical and emotional exercises. Just like a sailboat must trim its sails and change its course, you might need to tweak your regimen. As you begin to chart your triggers, you will learn more about your unique journey toward optimal health. If at any point in the four-week journey, your symptoms worsen significantly, please read the section on healing crises and decide whether or not it is appropriate for you to make some changes.

Make a commitment to yourself to learn how to manage your symptoms and have a more vibrant, healthy life. These recommendations can greatly impact every area of your health and well-being. Holistically managing your symptoms of herpes is not a quick fix; it is a process that takes time. This four-week program is a platform of health upon which you can build, but you must commit to *all* of the changes to get the best results. The goal here is to help you achieve a life in which herpes no longer triggers you, and you no longer trigger your herpes. Once you can get to a place where you are outbreak free for three months, you can begin, one by one, to reintroduce triggers.

In this step-by-step fashion, you will learn what your triggers truly are. This is why it is paramount to keep a journal of your progress charting your physical, mental, and emotional triggers. Once you learn this, you will be much more empowered to make decisions. Knowledge is power, and if you don't know what your triggers are, you will continue to feel powerless to your outbreaks. Learn what contributes to your outbreaks, and you can powerfully choose to take the risk.

Below you will discover the four-week quick-start self-care plan to begin your healing journey. The supplement and healing remedies guidelines are outlined at the end of this chapter. You will need these sections to fully participate in the quick-start program. I encourage you to make a weekly checklist to keep you better organized and to help you stay on track with your weekly goals. You can print one from www.PinkTent.com.

Quick-Start Self-Care Plan

Week One

1. Join our Pink Tent community and share your story at www. PinkTent.com.
2. Drink plenty of water! At least eight glasses, if not more, of spring or filtered water a day. Spring water is ideal.
3. Meditate for fifteen minutes first thing in the morning, during your lunch break, or just before bed. Wherever you can implement fifteen minutes of meditation in a twenty-four-hour period, do so.

4. Start eliminating foods high in arginine from your diet: nuts, seeds, chocolate, coffee (limit one cup per day). Please refer to page 143 for a complete list of foods high in arginine.

5. Decrease your sugar intake by removing foods high in sugar and empty in nutrients, including muffins, cookies, and cakes. For now replace sugar cravings with fresh fruit low in sugar like blueberries and apples.

6. Increase your consumption of vegetables, emphasizing green vegetables such as spinach, kale, and romaine lettuce.

7. Start supplementing your diet with the regimen outlined on 154-155: omega-3s, zinc, a multivitamin, D3, selenium and kelp. You may substitute garlic pills for a selenium supplement.

8. Implement two natural healing remedies into your regimen, found on pages 157-164. Start with two you have never tried before. Any two will do.

9. Reduce intense workouts and replace them with low-intensity workouts. This is a good time to sample gentle activities three to five times a week. Ideal exercises include yoga, long walks/hikes, and swimming. If you don't exercise, now is the time to start!

10. Remove extremes in temperatures from your environment. No more saunas, hot tubs, or hot yoga.

11. Start a healing journal, documenting what is and isn't working for you, how your body feels, and what your emotional and physical triggers are. Include dates and which week of the self-care plan you are in.

Week Two

1. Meditate daily. Incorporate an exercise from this book into your daily practice. Refer to the index for specific exercises.

2. Sleep is incredibly healing. If you can get eight hours or more of sleep, do so.

3. Drink eight or more glasses of water.

4. Continue to eliminate foods high in arginine and increase foods high in lysine: chicken and yogurt have some of the highest lysine values. Avoid low-fat yogurts because they tend to be high in sugar and artificial, toxic sweeteners.

5. Eliminate soda pop and replace it with carbonated water and lemon, lime, orange slices, or mint for flavor.
6. Continue taking your supplements daily.
7. Continue taking your natural healing remedies.
8. Continue decreasing any intense workouts.
9. Continue with your low intensity workouts including gentle activities such as yoga, long walks/hikes, and/or swimming three to five times a week.
10. Continue to journal and use your checklist.

Week Three

1. Meditate daily, and incorporate a different exercise from this book into your day.
2. Continue to sleep eight or more hours a day.
3. Continue to drink plenty of water.
4. If you haven't already completely eliminated foods high in arginine you *must* do so now. At this point, your diet should be high in lysine.
5. Be mindful of your sugar intake. Remember, excess sugar depletes your immunity and decreases your ability to heal.
6. Continue to take your supplement regimen.
7. If your symptoms are worsened, read the section on healing crises on page 26 and make a decision whether or not to change your routine. If you do discontinue your current remedies, replace them with two new ones.
8. Book an appointment with a bodyworker such as an acupuncturist, massage therapist, chiropractor, or energy worker. See the bodywork section for more ideas. If you are strapped for cash, research bodywork schools in your area; most often they have sliding scale programs.
9. Continue to implement low-intensity workouts, gentle activities such as yoga, long walks/hikes, and/or swimming three to five
. times a week.
10. Continue journaling and using your checklist.

Week Four

1. Meditate daily and include an exercise from this book. Implement this exercise daily.
2. Continue to sleep eight or more hours a day.
3. Decrease heavy metal exposure by following guidelines on pages 132-134.
4. Continue to drink plenty of water.
5. If you haven't already completely eliminated foods high in arginine you *must* do so now. At this point, your diet should be high in lysine and not arginine.
6. Maintain a diet low in sugar.
7. Continue to take all of your supplements.
8. If your symptoms are worsened read the section on healing crisis found on pages 26-27 and make a decision whether or not to change your routine. If you do discontinue your current remedies, replace them with two new ones.
9. Continue to implement low intensity workouts, gentle activities such as yoga, long walks/hikes, and/or swimming three to five times a week.
10. Continue journaling and using your checklist.
11. Increase your vegetable intake. A great way to do this is to weigh a week's worth of veggies in advance and eat a pound a week. Frozen is fine, but fresh is best.
12. Plan on cleansing during week five. This week, decide which cleanse is best for you. Review cleanse recommendations on pages 134-136.

Below is a herpes self-assessment so that you can begin to identify your unique imbalances and where you should focus your attention. I recommend that you do this before you begin the four-week plan.

Herpes Self-Assessment: Your Unique Imbalances

Please check with your doctor before adding new supplements.

Are you a vegetarian? You might not be getting enough good protein in your diet, and protein is needed to heal. Vegetarians are also at risk for copper toxicity. Vegetables are high in copper but low in zinc. Consider adding eggs to your diet and decreasing or eliminating seeds, which are too high in arginine (another trigger).

Do you have white spots on your nails? You might have a zinc deficiency. Zinc is important for wound healing and immunity. Start taking zinc.

Do you get your outbreaks at the same time every month? You might have a hormonal imbalance. Healthy omega-3s could help you to rebalance your hormones. (See the "Supplements and Herbs" section on pages 154-156). Find a good acupuncturist in your area to evaluate your condition.

Have you been on antibiotics several times in your life? This tells me two things: your immunity is depressed *and* your gut flora is probably out of balance. Take probiotics and do a cleanse.

Do you have sexual abuse in your past that you have never dealt with? Seek counseling and begin by doing the exercises on forgiveness (p. 50) and chakra healing (pages 71-78) contained in this book.

Do you crave sugar? This will greatly decrease your immunity! You could have a candida (yeast) overgrowth, heavy metal toxicity, or a mineral imbalance. Decrease your heavy metal exposure, cut the sugar, cut the fruit, do a cleanse, and add probiotics to your regimen.

Do you have dry skin or chapped lips? You're probably dehydrated! Drink more water and increase your omega-3s. Also, if you get herpes on your face, stay out of harsh wind and cold.

Do you frequent hot tubs, saunas, or hot yoga? You are too hot! Heat will make your outbreaks worse.

Do you love chocolate and nuts? These are high in the amino acid arginine. Remove these foods from your diet. Read more about food triggers in chapter six.

Do you commonly get vaginal yeast infections? Be sure to cut back on your sugar intake and add probiotics to increase your immunity.

Do you use a copper IUD (intrauterine device)? Copper IUDs can lead to a condition called copper toxicity. If this is occurring, the IUD could be further decreasing your immunity. The IUD could also be physically irritating to your cervix and increasing your outbreaks. Best solution? Remove the IUD and supplement with zinc to offset the delicate balance of copper and zinc in your system. (When copper is too high, zinc is too low.)

Do you have a bowel movement at least every day? If not, you are constipated and are definitely toxic. Do a colon cleanse and begin cleaning house.

Do you get outbreaks on your face when you are in the sun? The sunshine can trigger your outbreaks. Protect yourself from the sun with a hat and some natural sun block.

Do you eat protein shakes? These are high in arginine and could be contributing to your outbreaks.

Do you have a metallic taste in your mouth? Your body might be attempting to eliminate heavy metals. Begin to chelate out the metals with kelp and consider having a hair test for heavy metal toxicity.

Have you had trauma to the pelvic region, such as surgery or a car accident? Trauma to this region of the spine can cause inflammation and irritation of the sacral nerves. This is where genital herpes hides out and lies dormant. Trauma to the region can lead to an increase in outbreaks. Consider having some healing work done on this region. I recommend chiropractic or craniosacral therapy.

Supplements and Herbs

Below is a list of the top supplements to improve your health and more importantly, your ability to keep herpes at bay.

Please check with your doctor before implementing any of these suggestions.

Omega-3s: 2000 mg or more a day

Omega-3 fatty acids are one of my favorite compounds to talk about. When Americans went stir crazy with fat-free diets, they missed a key component of a healthy diet: *good* fats. Our diet is composed of proteins, carbohydrates, and fats. We need all of these in proper balance to achieve optimal health. Each cell in your body needs fat to function. All of your hormones, your brain, and your nervous system are mainly composed of fatty substance.

There are three main categories of unsaturated essential fatty acids: omega-3s, -6s and -9s. These fatty acids are aptly named by the location of their double bond at the third, sixth, and ninth position. Since the body cannot make these fats, they need to be obtained through the diet. In general, the standard American diet (SAD) is nearly devoid of the omega-3s, which are commonly found in fish, kelp, and nuts. Each of these fatty acids is important in the diet, but they need to be properly balanced in the system.

A typical American diet consists of too much omega-6s and not enough omega-3s. Reducing our omega-6's and increasing our omega-3s is one of the best things we can do for our overall health. Proper dietary changes and supplementation has been linked to cardiovascular health, decreased inflammation, decreased risk of breast cancer, improved immunity, rebalancing hormones, improved mental function, decreased depression, pain, and the list goes on and on.

If you have herpes, nuts and seeds are *not* a good source of omega-3s because of their high arginine values (hemp and flax seeds are an exception to the rule and are found to be beneficial). Supplement with fish oils, hemp, and flax. I take fish oils every day and eat two tablespoons of flax or hemp seeds straight up or on a salad. Fish oils have the added benefit of the hormone DHEA, which also has several healing properties including hormonal rebalancing, immune building, cardiovascular health, and brain health.

Zinc Chelate or Picolinate: 50 mg/day

Zinc is extremely important for immunity, skin health, and tissue repair. Most people are deficient in zinc, which is why it is often added to cough drops and lozenges. I noticed a huge difference in my herpes outbreaks once I consistently starting taking zinc as a supplement. To boot, my taste buds have become more alive. Zinc deficiency affects our ability to taste.

Multivitamin

There are several multivitamins on the market. Cheaper in this case is not better. Many of the cheap products are filled with binders and fillers. There is no way you can get everything in a multi, but at least you should get some basics, including calcium and magnesium. Be sure to supplement with at least 750 milligrams of calcium and 450 milligrams of magnesium. Did you know that after about the age of twenty-five, women need to have a calcium supplement because of our higher risk of osteoporosis (green leafy veggies are high in calcium and should help). Talk to your local holistic pharmacy or grocery rep to help steer you in the right direction.

Selenium: 200 mcg/day

Selenium is a trace mineral that is found in high concentrations in brewer's or nutritional yeast, seafood, and garlic. It reduces the risk of thyroid imbalance, heart disease, infertility, and preeclampsia. It is also an excellent immune builder and antioxidant.

Vitamin D3: 5000 mg/day

For years, medical experts thought that most people received enough vitamin D from the sun. Now they are discovering the importance of adding vitamin D as a supplement to our diet. Vitamin D is crucial for the absorption on calcium. It is an excellent immune builder and is required for proper bone health.

Kelp: 1500 mg/day

Word on the street is that most women have thyroid imbalances. *If you are taking medication for thyroid imbalance or have been diagnosed with hyperthyroidism or Hashimoto's disease, do not take kelp until you speak with your physician.*

Kelp does wonders to chelate out heavy metal toxins from our bodies. It also helps to balance our metabolism and to replace much-needed natural iodine in our bodies. The thyroid gland tends to store heavy metals, especially when iodine is not present. Before I added kelp to my regimen, my hair was falling out! You wouldn't notice it with my thick mane, but handfuls of hair were clogging our drain. Now my hair is staying in my head, and I have even lost a few extra pounds.

Kelp is high in iodine and several trace minerals. Most people think they are getting enough iodine from table salt, but it is the worst source of iodine and is hazardous to your health! In fact, it is a main culprit for raising blood pressure! Throw away the table salt and replace it with sea salt. Sea salt is all natural and actually contains trace minerals that are good for you. Our family loves to experiment with natural sea salts with different flavors and textures from around the world. Discover the healing properties of Himalayan salt or bamboo salt.

Healing Remedies

Some of these remedies interact with prescription drugs and should not be used by pregnant or breast-feeding mothers. Please contact your medical doctor before incorporating them into your herpes protocol.

As I have stated before, I believe that we must supplement our diets if we are to achieve optimal health. Once you have implemented the basic supplement regimen outlined above, you are ready to add some specific healing remedies to combat the herpes virus. What I love about natural remedies is that they are often inexpensive and readily available. This makes the potential return on investment in conducting huge alternative medical studies unattractive to big business. When stacked against the medical model, these remedies might fall short in the arena of scientific scrutiny, but where they shine is in their usage among healers across the ages. If you have never turned to alternative medicine, I encourage you to think outside of the box and try something new.

Start by implementing one or two remedies into your daily routine. Our primary goal here is to build up your immunity, the best defense for herpes. Be consistent in taking your regimen every day. Do not incorporate more than two internal healing remedies at a time because you will not know what is working. Give a remedy a couple of months before you give up on it. Natural medicine is not designed to give results overnight. It takes time for the body to respond to something natural. If after a few months you do not see any differences, try something new. In the meantime, focus on your overall personal wellness plan. Use the quick-start self-care plan outlined in this chapter to get you started in your wellness journey.

Just a quick note: many of these remedies will also work for outbreaks of shingles. I especially like to use colloidal silver gel and Lauricidin, a natural monolaurin supplement, for shingles.

Aloe vera: Aloe has been used for centuries as a remedy for many things including digestive disorders, high blood pressure, ulcers, inflammation, diabetes, low immunity, and skin conditions. I drink aloe vera every day in the form of Body Balance. For topical applications, the inner fillet of the plant can be applied to lesions to speed up the healing rate and soothe irritated, painful skin. Do not use creams with aloe, and only use gels that are close to 100 percent aloe. If you grow your own aloe plant, you can cut off a piece and filet it. Place the filet in the freezer and use it as needed, directly on the sore.

Astragalus: This ancient herb is often used in traditional Chinese medicine as an antidote to herpes. As an immune stimulator, it protects bone marrow cells. Be aware that astragalus is contraindicated with corticosteroids and immunosuppressive drug therapy.

Black tea: The tannins in black tea are both antiviral and anti-inflammatory. Steep some black tea in hot water for an hour. Allow the tea bag to cool. Place the warm or cold tea bag directly on the sore, and tear the bag to allow the tea to come into direct contact with the sore.

Burdock: This plant is a liver and blood cleanser that also relieves swollen glands.

Colloidal silver: Have you ever heard wealthy people referred to as "blue bloods"? This is a term based on the healing properties of silver.

Historically, wealthy people used silver utensils and "ate off of silver spoons." It was later discovered that this practice made them less susceptible to illness than their counterparts, the reason being that bits of silver from their utensils kept their immunity high. If they leeched too much silver into their system, they would literally turn blue.

Colloidal silver, as its name implies, is a silver suspension in a gel or liquid. It is one of my favorite remedies in my medicine chest. I use it every time my infant baby or my family has a hint of the flu or a cold. Use it during outbreaks as an antiviral. It is commonly used in medical clinics in third-world countries as their main antibiotic, antiviral, and antifungal. Do not take it daily longer than a couple of months because you could turn into a blue blood yourself. Yikes! Whenever I have an outbreak, I use it internally and use a gel topically. It does wonders to zap my sores.

WARNING: a higher parts per million (ppm) of silver in the liquid form does not mean that it is better. In fact, higher concentrations run the risk of creating toxicity in the body

Cornstarch and baking soda: Both of these ingredients act as drying agents and can help to dry out the sores and decrease itching. If your herpes is in an area that rubs, like the thighs, you can use cornstarch to decrease the friction and keep the area dry.

Dandelion: This plant supports the myelin sheath of nerves and is an excellent liver cleanser.

Epsom salt bath: If you are having a genital outbreak, a warm Epsom salt bath will both speed up the healing and decrease the itching.

Essential oils: There are several essential oils on the market that have been known to assist in pain management, skin healing, emotional balancing, and immune building. Some oils known to assist with healing herpes include tea tree oil (melaleuca), lavender, and lemon balm (Melissa). Be sure to dilute these oils in another oil carrier like vegetable oil or olive oil before applying them directly onto a sore. All of these oils have antiviral properties that directly attack the herpes virus. I use the brand name Young Living for my essential oils because they make such high-quality products.

Some oils also deliver therapeutic benefit when inhaled. Some of my favorite blends for a pick-me-up are Joy, Abundance, Tranquility, Peace, and Calm and Valor. I also highly recommend Raindrop Therapy (see the healing modality section on page 208 as a massage therapy to reduce stress, release toxins, and kill pathogens deep within the body.

Garlic: Garlic has been known for thousands of years for its healing properties. Its medicinal ingredient, allicin, along with its high sulfur content, minerals (especially selenium), and other phytochemicals make it an antiviral, antibacterial, antioxidant, and immune builder. It's also fantastic for the cardiovascular system. Garlic is inexpensive and very versatile. I cook with garlic almost every day. In order to save time, every four to six months I chop up a few heads of garlic in my Cuisinart, cover it in olive oil, and place it on the door of my refrigerator for future use. If you are not much of a cook, you can purchase it in pill form. If you can, choose the garlic brands that add mushroom blends for their immune-building properties, and take the pills daily. During outbreaks, increase your dosage. Keep the vampires away and use garlic every day!

Goldenseal: This anti-inflammatory immune builder is excellent for treating inflammation and damage to the mouth, eye, and throat.

Holy basil/tulsi: This is an herb that has been used in India for centuries. It is a revered plant in India, and in the Hindu tradition it is used for spiritual rituals and ceremony. Its use is varied, but my interest in its use is as an adaptogen, immune builder, and an antiviral for herpes. An adaptogen is a substance that helps to rebuild the adrenal glands without stimulating and irritating them. For many, it offers a boost of energy and mental clarity. As a result, many people use it in place of caffeine (a detrimental substance for a newly diagnosed herpes sufferer). You can drink this as a tea or as a supplement.

Ice and cold water: For pain relief, use a bag of ice or a bag of frozen veggies directly on a sore. You can also run cold water over your genitals for five to ten minutes. If urinating is painful, you might want to urinate in the shower or in a bath with a small amount of water.

Lauricidin: I recently discovered this all-natural formula and am thrilled to introduce it to you. For years, I have recommended the use of coconut oil due to its antiviral properties. I, along with Dr. Weil, now recommend Lauricidin in place of it. Lauricidin is the brand name for a formula that contains very high levels of monolaurin, the same medicinal compound found in coconut oil, but in much higher doses. The CDC (Center for Disease Control) studied this supplement back in the early eighties and discovered that it did in fact kill the herpes virus on contact. Lauricidin can be taken daily to improve immunity, and it can be made into a cream to apply topically to herpes sores. This all-star fat molecule has also been shown to be beneficial with HSV, shingles, autoimmune disorders, Lyme's disease, MERSA, autism, candida, acne, and several other disorders. The recommended dosage for an otherwise healthy adult is one scoop three times a day; at the onset of herpes symptoms or during outbreaks this dosage can be doubled. For topical use for herpes and shingles, add one scoop to two ounces of hot water, stir occasionally as it cools, and apply several times a day.

Lemon balm (Melissa officinalis): This herb is part of the mint family. It is an antiviral found in several herpes products including oils, tinctures, ointments, and healing formulas. One study found that lesions healed in half the time when ointments containing lemon balm were applied to a sore five times a day. It is an excellent nerve relaxer and nervous system tonic. It is much stronger if it is fresh, and you can grow it yourself and make a daily tea with it. Dried lemon balm is of little therapeutic use. Some have found that if you apply it as an oil directly on a sore, it will speed up the healing process.

Licorice Root and DGL (deglycyrrhizinated licorice): This is known to support the immune system and the adrenal glands. Reports indicate that it is effective against HSV-1, but HSV-2 effectiveness is unclear. Do not take if you suffer from high blood pressure.

L-lysine: Lysine is an amino acid that has been shown to be low in people with herpes. Many herpes sufferers swear by this natural remedy. This supplement can be found in salves, or it can be taken internally. If you would like to supplement your diet with this, I suggest doing so *only* during outbreak modes. Taken daily, the delicate balance of lysine and arginine in the body could be set too far out of balance. Eating a diet high in lysine and low in arginine is a safer daily alternative. During outbreaks, take 2mg of Lysine every four hours, till symptoms subside.

Medicinal mushrooms: mushrooms have been used to fight diseases for over a millennium in parts of Asia. The polysaccharides found in mushrooms have been researched since the 1960s for their medicinal properties. Mushrooms are known to be antiviral, antibacterial, antibacterial, antiparasitic, antidiabetic, anti-inflammatory, heart healthy, and immune building. Some herpes experts consider shiitake mushrooms to be the queen of the mushroom world. Your can either eat them or supplement with extracts or pills. Either way, go for organic because mushrooms tend to soak up toxicities from their environment.

Olive leaf extract: This extract comes from the olive tree. Reports have shown that this remedy is successful in treating over fifty reported pathogens including HSV-1 and HSV-2. It is an antiviral, antibacterial, antifungal, antioxidant, and anti-inflammatory. It lowers blood pressure, lowers blood sugars, and reduces clotting. It can be taken internally and can also be used topically on active lesions.

Prunella vulgaris: This herb is often used in Chinese medicine. It has antiviral, antimicrobial, and antioxidant properties and has traditionally been used in folk medicine to cure ailments in China and Asia. Some experts believe that the rosmarinic acid and triterpenoid found in this herb could benefit those with HSV-1 and HSV-2.

Rescue remedy: This is a blend of Bach flower essences I have found to be extremely powerful in calming the nervous system. Take this formula internally any time you feel anxious or in overwhelm, and it will help you to calm you down.

Red clover: This is a general tonic for the nerves, a blood cleanser, and a liver cleanser.

Seaweeds: Our soil might be depleted of minerals, but the sea has an abundance of them. Seaweeds contain an amazing amount of vitamins, minerals, and phytonutrients. For centuries seaweeds have been consumed in Asia, where they experience very little heart disease and cancer as a culture. Red marine algae has been touted as a herpes-healing food, but it is often sourced from polluted waters. I would stay clear of red marine algae supplements and use other seaweeds instead. You can add wakame and dulse seaweeds to your food, or you can drink my favorite, healthy, yummy "vitamin in a bottle," Body Balance from Life Force International (www.lifeforce.net enrollment #20450958 or call 1(800) 531-4877). It is composed of nine different sea vegetables, so you can have the benefit of phytochemicals from several sources. I drink it every day to keep my immunity in tiptop shape.

Siberian ginseng (Eleutherococcus senticosus): Ginseng increases energy, vitality, mental clarity, and immunity. It also strengthens over-stressed adrenal glands. Beware if you are on blood thinners, sedatives, or heart medications.

St. John's wort: Hypericin is the active ingredient known to act as an antidepressant, antiviral, and energy booster. This may be contraindicated if you are on any prescription drugs. It also causes photosensitivity, so wear sunscreen.

Taheebo or pau d'arco: This is a powerful medicinal herb originally from South America. It has been reported to help with diabetes, candida, cancer, decreased immunity, HIV/AIDS, liver disorders, blood purification, and many other things. It is high in minerals and can be consumed as a tea. I personally use the Taheebo from Life Force International (Call 1(800) 531-4877) enrollment #20450958). You can place it in hot water as a tea, drink it directly, or sip it diluted in water throughout the day.

Vitamin C: Vitamin C, also known as ascorbic acid, is a powerful antioxidant and immune builder. It also plays a significant role in wound healing because it is required for the synthesis of collagen (a protein found in flesh and connective tissue). Linus Pauling, a scientist who won a Nobel Prize for his work with vitamin C, suggested using megadoses of vitamin C for conditions such as the common cold and cancer. If you choose to supplement vitamin C in your diet, consider using Ester-C® because it is a more absorbable form. If you experience abdominal pain or diarrhea, back off a bit on the vitamin C.

Vitamin E: If you are left with a scar or a reddening of the skin after your lesion has healed, I recommend applying some vitamin E on your sore. There are experts who believe that scarring can impact the electrical circuitry of the nervous system, especially if it is a midline scar. This means that a scar, running across the center of your body, i.e., a horizontal scar, will interfere with your nervous system. Usually collagen fibers come together in a clean webbing or woven pattern. Scar tissue is a jagged or torn collection of collagen fibers that block the natural flow of the body's electrical circuitry. Essentially, when you heal your scar, you will heal a blockage or impasse of energy within that specific area. If you have had any surgeries or other scars that are midline in your body, I would also recommend you heal them with the daily application of vitamin E and massage the fibers so that they release the jagged fibers and come back into their natural woven pattern. There are several sources that work, but almond oil and jojoba are two of my favorites.

Specific Remedies for Oral Herpes

Gum-Omile: This infant teething oil works wonders. It is made from almond oil, willow bark extract, chamomile flowers extract, essential oil of clove bud, and vitamin E oil. The clove oil takes the sting out while the other ingredients have anti-inflammatory and healing properties.

Salt-water rinse: A simple, inexpensive home remedy for expediting the healing of herpes in the mouth is to dilute a teaspoon of salt in eight ounces of warm water. Salt water improves healing time. Salt kills off bacteria and viruses and is also very soothing for the skin.

Taheebo: Taheebo is extremely helpful for oral herpes. I have found it to significantly speed up the healing rate. Apply it directly on the sore and also take it internally.

Vita-Myr: This is a high-end mouthwash, made up of the following:

Clove: anti-inflammatory, antiseptic

Distilled water: Most mouthwash uses alcohol as a base. This is very irritating to the gums and soft tissue in the mouth. This mouthwash uses distilled water as a base. As a side benefit, this mouthwash is excellent for helping to repair symptoms of gum disease.

Folic acid: anti-inflammatory

Myrrh oil: anti-inflammatory and immune stimulant

Zinc picolinate: reduces healing time

EIGHT

Learning to Love Yourself and Others

True love is no game of the faint-hearted and the weak; it is born of strength and understanding.

—MEHER BABA

We Are Gems

I had just completed my first year in chiropractic practice and was feeling worn down from the trials and tribulations that go hand and hand with being a new business owner. Despite it all, I had survived and was feeling proud of my accomplishments. Within a month of celebrating my one-year anniversary at Expression of Life, PC, I received an announcement from my dear friend, Shan, who was getting married. I was ecstatic for him, for he had found the love of his life.

While I experienced immense joy for Shan, with it came heartache. There was nothing I wanted more in my life than to meet the man I would spend my life with. What was the matter with me? Why was it that I was still all alone? While my kitties, Maverick and Jesse, were my warm companions at the end of the day, I was eager to have something a bit less furry to come home to. Salsa dancing with friends on Friday nights always ended the same way: alone in my one-bedroom apartment surrounded by affirmations and journals expressing my desire to find a mate.

A 1920s vintage green zircon platinum ring, mounted in diamond-studded filigree, changed everything for me. I can still envision it behind the glass of my favorite antique jewelry store in Boulder, Colorado, called Classic Facets. Now, mind you, I have always had a thing for circa 1920s jewelry, but no other piece had captured my heart and mind like that green zircon ring. I would stroll down Pearl Street on my lunch breaks just to place it on my finger, dreaming about owning it some day. It made me feel beautiful and elegant. Dreams of the majestic ring would visit me in the night. Who had owned it? What was her life like? Did her green rock shimmer on the dance floor as she playfully danced the Charleston with her loving husband?

As my mind wrestled with my heart, I made one last phone call to my mother to ask for her opinion. For the record, she had a hand in developing my taste for antique jewelry at such a young age. In my box of treasures, I had already acquired heirloom pieces that were given to me at significant stages of my life. To her, the dream was not so crazy. She had visited me several months before and had examined the ring under a loop to determine its validity.

Then one rainy Friday afternoon, after sitting in meditation, I slipped into my comfy, tattered jeans, placed my checkbook in my purse, and set out on a quest to seriously consider purchasing the ring. Before I made any irrational decision, I knew that it would be best to have a full tummy, so I treated myself to a late brunch. It was an outlandish, crazy idea for a woman who had just started a private practice and was up to her head in alligators with student debt to even consider buying such a ring. However, there was one thing: I did have a little nest egg of savings. It was not the golden nest egg I would have liked to have accumulated, but it was a small safety blanket to weather life's unknown surprises. I promised myself that if I were ever going to take the risk and buy the ring, I would do it with cash and not with credit. The cost of the ring amounted to nearly all of my savings, more than my month's pay.

I was pretty certain it was the day to take the plunge. I had discovered something special. Although I had no man in my life, I had myself, family, friends, and two precious sidekick kitties. I had spent hours and hours hiking, meditating, journaling, running, and in solitude. The silence of my alone time had infused me with a deep love and appreciation for who I was and how I showed up in the world. I found out the greatest gift of all: I was my very own best friend and partner. I realized that I did not need to find love in partnership; instead, I could discover it from within. I discovered that I did not need external love from another. I realized that there was absolutely nothing wrong with me, and if I waited for a guy to give me all that I wanted, rather then giving it to myself, i.e., buying the ring, I might never receive it. I also realized that I immensely enjoyed time with myself. If you can be with yourself and be happy, then I can almost guarantee that others will find enjoyment in spending time with you.

It was time I placed a line in the sand and married myself. On May 20, 2005, I purchased the most spectacular, eye-catching, sparkling green zircon platinum ring I'd ever seen and placed it on my finger. I later discovered that another woman who had been admiring the piece came into the shop to purchase it only an hour after I had. It was not her time, though; it was mine. Does the universe have a plan for us? I think so! From this act of celebration and commitment to love myself, I surrendered to God's plan for me. I believe that this act was a great milestone for my healing journey.

By the summer of 2009, Richard and I were shopping for engagement rings. Within a few weeks of shopping for rings, I noticed that my zircon ring had lost some of its sparkle. There were a few diamond studs within the filigree that had fallen out from the side of the ring. In order to fix the ring, I had to send it out for a repair. I was heartbroken, for I had worn that ring every day since its purchase and felt completely naked without it. Over a month passed by until we got word that the ring was not repairable. My ring was sent around the country, hopping from ring specialist to ring specialist in hopes of finding someone who could repair it. Apparently, the problem was that a previous owner had tried to cut corners on a repair by using white gold instead of platinum. Unfortunately for me, when you put two dissimilar metals together, they can eat away at one another, weakening their bond. I was told it was as if my ring had cancer! The only way to save the ring was to make a mold of it, disassemble it, and rebuild it, a very expensive process. My disassembled gem still sits in our safe as a project for the very near future.

Later in June, my gorgeous green zircon ring took the back seat to a beautiful, sparkling diamond ring. I needed to make room for Richard's love in my life. Our wedding band was gifted to us from my mother, who wore the piece as an accent to her vintage sapphire ring. My parents are still married after forty-three years, and my mother's band sits below the 1920s-style engagement ring that Richard gave me. Richard still tells me that the ring he gave me signifies his heart, and any time he is away from me, I can always look down at my ring. So, now I have a wedding band signifying the stability of my parent's union upholding my engagement ring. Both Richard and I are certain that our love will stand the test of time.

Are You Open to Love?

If you want to attract a healthy, loving mate, start by being healthy and loving to yourself. We must learn to love ourselves, and through this we will radiate and attract love into our lives. I truly believe that I found Richard because we both had learned to love ourselves. When we came together, we uplifted one another to a higher platform. We had done the hard work in order to reap the benefit of grace. Our union was easy and natural because we knew what we wanted and were able to identify and acknowledge it.

Richard's love was like none I had ever experienced. In his presence, I felt like we could climb any mountain. I knew that he would be there for me through both good and bad times. He was the person with whom I wanted to weather the storms in life. He soon became my lover and best friend. Together we were stronger than we could ever be apart. Life flowed easily and effortlessly together, and for the first time in my life I could totally surrender and let go of the reigns. I trusted that if I faltered, he would be there to catch me.

But believe me, after I returned home from Nepal and reentered my life as a young, single woman, I had a lot of frogs to kiss before I found my prince. Over those years, I learned a great deal about myself and the men

I was attracting into my life. Most of these men were good-looking, self-absorbed, and emotionally unavailable. Boulder is a magnet for the Peter Pan men of the world, all play and no commitment. I had to find my voice first and discover that I deserved to be cherished. Who cared if these men had abs of steel or that they could have modeled for *GQ*! At the end of the day, none of that really mattered. So, for the next several years, I kept my priorities focused on becoming a doctor and gave up on finding Mr. Right, for I would date Mr. Right for Now.

What happened over all of those years in regards to dating? It is my opinion that I was not ready to attract my soul mate. My having herpes put up more of a barrier than I realized at the time. I kept myself at arm's length in fear of being hurt or having to show my vulnerability. Once I became a doctor, my focus went from my studies to my patients. I was an independent warrior and did not *need* a man even though I wanted one. I will never forget the time I brought a guy I was dating to my beautiful office. I never saw him again, and I don't think it was the first time I intimidated men with my level of success. I was a feminist at heart who believed that women could do it all. What I was not being true to was the desire to find a man who could take care of me—*could*—if I wanted him to. "Choice" was the key word for me.

I was thrilled when I brought my now husband to the office for the first time, and within a few weeks he showed up with a tool belt and a drill to fix a broken chiropractic table for me. That was sexy hot for me! My barriers of fear were softening.

At one point, before I met Richard, I was bawling my eyes out to my mother on the phone, and I asked her if I was demanding way too much. She assured me that the right guy was out there and that I needed to keep my head held high and to have faith. Although I doubted her advice, within months I met the man I am proud to say is my husband, best friend, and father of our baby girl. We attract what we are ready for, and until I met Richard, I had not done my homework. In other words, I was fearful of heartbreak and therefore put up a wall as to not let anyone in.

Like attracts like, right? Ladies, you have to go on the inner journey and learn how to totally love yourself, the whole package you present to another. We are by nature attractors. Many of us don our warrior gear on a daily basis so that we can appear strong and able in a male-dominated world. We are not meant to be *doing* all the time; we are meant to be *being*.

Once I got this on a cellular level and cleared the layers of self-limiting beliefs and disappointments from my consciousness, I was a clear, attracting magnet. I tuned my radio signal for finding my perfect mate on high, and the signal was as clear as ever. Within a month of doing an intense healing session on releasing the past and being open to the future, I met my husband.

Feeling Sexy and Deserving of Love

We are meant to know and own our inner goddess. Historically, men have squelched our power, intuition, inner beauty, and strength. Please, don't let herpes rob you of your strengths as a woman. Be proud of the freedom you have to express your inner goddess, for not all women around the world have this opportunity. Don't lock yourself away in a world of isolation. Surround yourself with a community of powerful women who will love and support you. Allow yourself to love deeply and to feel sexy. Walk the catwalk! Go to Victoria's Secret and buy yourself a new pair of sexy panties.

Once you start feeling sexy again and you are ready to enter into new partnerships, don't be surprised if your self-love quotient is challenged. Months would go by without an outbreak, but whenever I began dating someone new, my herpes symptoms often went berserk and I began feeling insecure again. It was as if on a deep, subconscious level, I did not feel deserving of love. My body would create the herpes symptoms so that I would be forced to "be with" my darkest secrets. On some level I was asking myself if this person would *actually* stick around despite my herpes? It wasn't until I met Richard that I realized how I was so scared to let a man into my life. Initially my outbreaks increased when I met him, but after several months of surrendering to his love, the outbreaks ceased.

I later shared this story with a patient of mine, Jane, who was experiencing an increase in symptoms with her new partner, Tom. She was wondering why, after thirty years of occasional outbreaks, her symptoms were increasing in frequency. Nothing else in her life had changed, and Tom was aware of her herpes status. I asked her if she felt deserving of his love. She was taken aback by the question. I challenged her to go inward and ask herself if on some level she was challenging Tom's commitment and love for her. I told her my theory was that since she thought Tom was *the* guy, she was left in a more vulnerable place and therefore taking more risks by staying in a relationship with him. If he could not handle the frequent outbreaks, she would not have to let his love in. Men and women do this all the time to self-sabotage a meaningful and healthy relationship. Our intimate relationships act as mirrors for all of our insecurities. I do believe that the power of self-love can immensely contribute to our healing. Jane agreed to do some meditation and self-inquiry on my theory, but felt that it had some validity for her life. This was not the first time I had seen this pattern before. Let Jane's story and mine serve as examples for how our thoughts can contribute to our symptoms.

Herpes allows us to surrender time and time again into a deeper commitment to self-love. We all feel vulnerable when we enter into a new relationship, whether we have herpes or not. Maybe your potential partner also has some shadows to reveal to you. I certainly took a risk with Richard when he told me of his sobriety. Was I willing to enter into a partnership knowing that alcohol had nearly ruined his life?

True intimacy starts with a thin veil of vulnerability. To live and love requires us to take chances. It is your vulnerability that will lead you to greater depths of intimacy, and herpes gifts you with the opportunity to dive deep into transparency in partnership. People are hungry for true connections. It takes a great deal of energy to hide behind your past. Trust yourself and your feelings. I too felt vulnerable when I told Richard about my herpes. Feel the fear and do it anyway—it's worth it!

My First "Talk" after Diagnosis

One of the first major milestones in my journey with herpes was having the infamous "talk" for the first time, after my diagnosis. This first intimate talk was definitely the hardest. I broke all the rules!

- I did NOT tell my boyfriend before things were rolling with passion.
- I did NOT give him time to make a decision whether or not to move forward in our relationship.
- I did NOT remain calm and detached.

Oops! Truth be told, things were steamy and passionate in the bedroom when I stopped and told him I had something to tell him. By the look on his face, he might have thought I was terminal or maybe an axe murderer. Why was I stopping things so abruptly?

I took a deep breath and peered deep into his soul, wondering if our love could triumph. I fought back the tears pooling at the corners of my eyes. My stomach churned with fear, shame, and a deep wounded sadness.

The floodgates released, and my voice quivered as I shared with him my deepest, darkest secret in the world. I had herpes! Once I uttered these words, I braced for rejection and was shocked by the warm embrace.

He was not that familiar with herpes, and I wasn't equipped with the arsenal of information I now have. He lovingly gazed into my eyes, wiped my tears, and said we would take this journey together. He held me as waves of uncontrollable shaking crashed over me, as I processed the scars that herpes had left on my soul.

At such an early stage in our relationship, divulging this secret brought Jack and me closer together. Instead of pulling us apart, "the Talk" created a foundation of trust we could then build upon. Our level of intimacy deepened as a result of my sharing. For the first time in my life, I opened a door inside me and allowed the skeletons in my closet to see the light of day.

It was cathartic for me to let it all out. My transparency felt freeing, and at the same time there was an enormous amount of personal growth work that was set into motion.

Practice Makes Perfect

Each time I had "the Talk," I felt more and more confident about the outcome, and about myself. By the time I started dating Richard, my now husband, and shared my story with him, I didn't even cry. I was nervous, of course, but I had experienced such positive outcomes in the past that I figured my chances of him understanding me were good, if not great.

I think the more confident you are about what you bring to the table in a relationship, the less and less herpes affects your life. Richard's reaction was positive. He asked a few questions about what the virus was and how it might interfere with us as a couple. I explained that there was a chance that I could transmit the virus to him, regardless of how careful we were, because of asymptomatic shedding.

He too was willing to absorb the risk with me and to take the next step in our relationship. We then shared our dating and sexual histories with each other. At one point in the conversation, I told him that if he had any other questions about herpes, I wanted him to ask me.

At that point in the relationship it was evident that we were falling madly in love with one another, and herpes did not even seem like the slightest issue. If that was all the baggage that I brought from past relationships, he was thrilled having dated enough women to realize that I was a gem. Within six months we were engaged!

Over time, having "the Talk" does became easier and easier.

The Fear of Rejection

Occasionally, I hear stories of rejection, but although rejection can be devastating, it doesn't have to be. Most people report having positive experiences with "the Talk." Never forget that you are not your herpes. Repeat after me: "I am not my herpes."

Again, one more time with gusto, "I am not my herpes." You are a person who lives with it. The fear of rejection is a valid concern for a person preparing to share her story of herpes with a potential partner. The first thing I must say is that if the person rejects you, *you* are not the one being rejected: herpes is. This is a very difficult distinction you must make in this circumstance. You are not your herpes, and you are not your past.

We all enter into relationships with what we hope to be an overnight bag of luggage, but for most it is a whole stack, high and precarious, ready to topple over. I have slimmed my baggage down over the years and still have not been able to totally clear my past in each and every moment I'm alive, which is my intention.

If we could truly do this we could create magic in every breath, because everything in essence would be cleansed of preconceptions. Maybe we could see the beauty in every moment as a gift from God. When we are truly present, there is no past and no future.

Never bring a past rejection into the future you are moving into. If you are ever rejected, take a deep breath and move forward. Don't allow the rejection to thwart your confidence in sharing your story with future partners. The best thing you can say to yourself is *"Next!"* Keep your heart open to love!

Why Waiting to Have "the Talk" Is Not the Best Idea

The longer you wait to share your secret, the harder it becomes. Over time, we begin to make up stories in our heads, and often they're not about the desired outcome but about the worst-case scenario. I have spoken with people who have harbored the secret of herpes for years, suffering in silence.

When I first began openly sharing my personal journey with herpes, I found that people would open up to me and want help. By standing in my own power as a woman, doctor, and healer, I gave them permission to stand in theirs. Authenticity is the new celebrity! Carrying our emotions in an airtight container weighs heavily on our hearts and has the potential to make us ill. Our emotions are meant to flow through us.

One day I was speaking at a women's entrepreneurial luncheon, and I was asked to give my thirty-second pitch. My heart began to race, and perspiration moistened my hands. In that moment I had a very important decision to make. I could play it safe and pitch my business as a chiropractor specializing in energy-based medicine and nutrition, or I could get naked (or so it felt) and announce that my specialty was in using my personal journey with herpes to assist other women with herpes to heal.

It was a pivotal moment for me because up until that time, I had never announced to a group of women that I have herpes. When I did, the shock in the room felt palpable, and I am certain that other women could not believe what I had just said. But I decided to be authentic and that, in and of itself, was liberating.

At the end of the meeting, an older woman waited for an extended period of time to talk to me. I sat down and was knee-to-knee with her while she shared her story of herpes for the first time in thirty years. As you can imagine, the tears came rolling down her face after years and years of suppression. There we met, soul to soul, as if there was no one else in the room.

We created a sacred space in that moment that allowed her to open up, quite possibly in ways that she never had to anyone but me—a complete stranger! This sixty-four-year-old woman had been diagnosed thirty years ago and had been able to keep it a secret from her husband, whom she had been with the whole time. She said that she had not cheated on him, but that the symptoms showed up for the first time after they had been married.

She explained how her outbreaks were severe enough that it was painful for her to sit down. I asked if she had been intimate with her husband since her diagnosis and she said yes, but that she would blame her period or a headache to keep him at arm's length during outbreaks. I was shocked to hear that she had two grown children and had shared a bed with a man for thirty years without ever telling him.

Her inspiration for telling me her story was that she had recently been divorced and was still getting outbreaks, and was scared to death to date. We set up an appointment the following week, and my level of confidence in helping other people grew a bit more. Here was a woman who suffered dearly in silence. Who else was out there hiding in the shadows? I was being called to shine a light on them and to radiate my own joy.

If you have been hiding in the shadows, it is time to share your story. The longer you wait, the longer you will suffer. In the end, I'm certain that you'll feel as if a huge weight has been lifted from your heart, and that you'll literally feel lighter. I can't promise that you won't shed tears, and in fact I encourage you to allow them to come if they do.

When Would YOU Want to Be Told?

One beautiful, sunny day in Boulder, I was taking a hike with my friend Nina and my dog Samantha. We were engaged in a great conversation about herpes and its implications. I was very pregnant at the time, and pacing was slow up the long gradual dirt trail to Sanitas Mountain.

It was a busy day on the trail, and as such, I didn't notice the footsteps of a woman behind us eavesdropping on our conversation. She must have been following us for some time because our conversation had already changed topics before the woman behind us excused herself. "Were you talking about herpes?" she asked. I told her that in fact we were, and that I was writing a book on the topic and collecting women's stories.

She proceeded to share her best friend's experience with dating someone with herpes. Her friend had fallen in love and become engaged to a stripper in Las Vegas. Within weeks of the wedding, his fiancée revealed her herpes status. She had been too embarrassed to tell him, and couldn't keep her secret any longer.

He was so hurt by her inability to confide in him that he felt that this lack of trust and integrity was enough to break off the engagement and cancel the wedding. If only she had told him early on in their courtship, he said that he could have accepted it. He was comfortable with her being a stripper, but secrets like herpes were totally unacceptable!

When I heard the story, my heart went out to the two of them. It is a great example of how you must put your heart and soul on the line before you enter the sacred contract of marriage, with trust being the foundation for everything. My reaction was that of sadness.

If only this woman had had a support system and a community to confide in. Talking about herpes is the first step in learning how to deal with it. This story also teaches us that herpes doesn't have to be a deal breaker, although in this case it was. Let your partner decide what he is willing to accept in the relationship. His answer might surprise you. Be curious. Before you open up to someone, imagine yourself in his shoes.

When would you want to be told? I don't think you need to divulge on your first date, unless, of course, things get hot and heavy. Be responsible, ethical, and compassionate toward yourself and others. FYI, there have been several lawsuits about the transmission of herpes to an uninfected person. An upstanding citizen does not need this fear of litigation to encourage her to divulge her secret of having herpes, but we live in a litigious society so it is important that you be aware of this.

The Dos and the Don'ts

Feel your fear and do it anyway!

—SUSAN JEFFERS

I first shared my secret with Kevin, the guy who gave it to me. This may or many not be appropriate for you. I then turned to my friend Peter, and then to my sister, mother, and best friend back home. There wasn't a whole lot of thinking about how I would tell them; I just did.

This may not come as naturally for you as it did for me. I tend to be the kind of woman who needs to talk things through in order to better understand my predicament or my suffering. I have discovered over the years that I process a lot of stuff by verbalizing it to a person who is really able to listen. This is one of the most important things to think about before sharing your story.

For many women, it's good to start with a best friend. Best friends often have the ability to listen without judgment. Don't be surprised if your story leads her (or him) to open up more profoundly to you. It's like a Pandora's box of connections.

Below I have identified some best general practices when preparing to have "the Talk."

Do...

Have integrity and have "the Talk" before you have exposed your partner in any way. Trust is the foundation of any relationship, and if you wait until after you might have exposed someone, it's all downhill from there! Trust is one of the most challenging things to repair when it has been lost. The earlier you have "the Talk," the better.

Celebrate your partnership. Take a moment to embrace what has transpired up until this very moment for the two of you. Create a space for your partner to share anything else that has been on his or her mind. Maybe your partner is right in sync with you to move forward, or maybe this is not the case, for unrelated reasons. Is the spark there? Are there red flags for either of you? "the Talk" gives you the chance to review what is really going on beyond the surface. If things are going great, it is a perfect time to acknowledge the other person for what he or she means to you.

Create a connection with cold sores. You might be wondering what I mean by this, but the reality is, there is an incredibly large percentage of people who either have cold sores or know of friends and family members with HSV1 (the herpes virus that causes cold sores). Herpes, in general, has a stigma, but if you start the conversation with

"Do you ever get cold sores or know of any family or friends who get cold sores?" this allows your partner to personally connect with herpes without making a negative judgment right away. When you can destigmatize herpes in this way, it will hopefully lessen the charge around the conversation.

Ask for confidentiality. It is paramount that you trust whomever you choose to tell first. Ask if the other person has time at that moment to share, and ask for confidentiality. This will displace some fear of your secret being spread. You can intuit who can hold this space for you, but I do suggest you verbalize it.

Speak directly from your heart. Each and every person will have a unique story to share. It's totally normal to tear up or cry while sharing your story. Allow yourself to feel your feelings. Get knee to knee and heart to heart, take a deep breath, and share.

Tell a friend or family member before you tell your partner. It will take some of the burden off of the conversation. Once you have told a friend or family member, you will be one step closer to telling a partner. A great way to ease into this is to role-play with a friend whom you have already told. Sometimes this is enough to take some of the charge out of "the Talk." Just knowing one other person knows about your struggles is extremely comforting.

Learn more about herpes. Get the facts and learn how you can manage your symptoms naturally. Knowledge is power, and it will help you build your confidence and allow you and your partner to assess your risks of transmission. If you have recently been diagnosed, your first task is to learn more about herpes, your body, your triggers, and how to manage your symptoms naturally. This in and of itself might seem like a tremendous load to carry. Use the resources and references in this book to help you navigate any questions that might arise. This book is full of great resources, even if you aren't a woman. You might even want to have this book nearby when you are ready to have "the Talk." Lending this book to your partner might help him or her to get better educated, to make an informed decision, and to learn how better to support you.

Get tested. Find out if your partner has ever been tested specifically for herpes, and for that matter, other STDs that would put you at risk. Please note that herpes is not included in a standard STD panel. You should also be up-to-date on STD screenings. For some, this is the perfect time in the relationship for you both to be screened. Don't forget that there are things like hepatitis and HIV out there as well. Herpes has given you the opportunity to get clear about who you want to be with. Risks exist for both parties, and this is the perfect excuse to learn what you are getting into. If your partner has not been tested for herpes or other STDs, now is the time. Health is something you should cherish and not take for granted. Some partners will be well versed in herpes, and others will be absolutely clueless. Despite your partner thinking he is negative for herpes, find out for sure with a blood test. That way, if test results reveal that you both have the same strain of herpes, you can't pass it back and forth to one another. What freedom! After you have all of your test results back and your partner decides to move forward in the relationship, have an open conversation about risks. Get clear on the worst-case scenario for the two of you and go from there.

Give your partner space. Once you share your story with your potential partner, I encourage you to give him or her the space to choose the appropriate next step. Some people will need time to process the new information you have given them, and yet they will not ask for it for fear of hurting your feelings. For some, the conversation of genital herpes is a new one. It can be overwhelming at first, and it is important to sort out the emotions from the facts and risks involved. Giving your partner time to process the new information will allow space to integrate associated feelings and clearly sort out how he or she wants to proceed.

Be willing to press the pause button on the relationship. Some people might feel more comfortable getting to know you better before diving into the next level of intimacy. This is actually a very healthy place from which to come. Some of the best relationships are founded on strong friendships. Pulling back the reigns on intimacy or pausing for a bit might actually make your connection stronger in the long run.

Give your partner information. Maybe your partner needs to peruse a Web site like www.pinktent.com or www.ashastd.org or www.cdc.gov. Purchase some books about herpes and make them available to your partner. Seeing the facts from reputable sources might allow your partner to feel more confident in the decision that he or she makes.

Turn your cell phone off. Need I say more?

Don't...

Dramatize things or go into victim mode, because this only complicates things. If you go into hysterics over this talk, your partner may become even more unsettled. Dramatizing your status might place your partner in a position of total fear of contracting the virus, especially if your partner is new to "the Talk."

Get defensive. If your partner needs time to process this, it doesn't mean he or she won't come around. Believe me, you want your partner to understand the risk of entering into the partnership before engaging. You would feel horrible if you transmitted herpes and your partner never understood what that meant.

Share your herpes status right in the heat of passion. This is probably one of the most common mistakes. In the heat of passion, no one is thinking clearly. Doing this places your partner in a precarious position and does not allow sufficient time to make a level-headed, informed decision about whether or not to move forward.

Make it all about you. Use this time to provide your partner with support and information. Your story is important, but "the Talk" is more about opening up a dialogue for your partner to speak. Ask engaging questions about your partner and how he or she might feel.

Find out if he or she has ever had an STD. Find out more about his or her sexual history. Don't make it a litany of questions, but be sure that your conversation is balanced.

Choose a public place to have the "Talk". Create the right space to share your story. Be in a quite space, in a secluded area of a park, or making tea in the comfort of your own home. Create enough room to breathe, and make sure you're also in a space that will support your partner's reactions and responses to the information.

If you follow these simple guidelines, you will set yourself up for success. Remember, there is no such thing as perfection when you are sharing your story. Be yourself and try not to be attached to the outcome of your sharing.

Taking the Charge Out of Your Story—An Exercise

The initial shock of a herpes diagnosis can leave you feeling raw and exposed. It feels like your life is tumbling down around you. Many sufferers go into a state of depression while their emotions whirl about them. These initial feelings associated with future outbreaks can become locked deep within the body.

When we prepare ourselves for "the Talk," sometimes these raw emotions can surface once again. It's as if the cells remember the trauma of the initial crisis, even though our lives appear to have moved on. As a chiropractor, I have had patients re-experience all sorts of memories from their past. This tends to occur when their bodies are ready to release their story and enter a deeper level of healing. Here is an exercise if you find yourself in a position of heightened emotions when you attempt to share your story.

1. *Find some quiet time and space for you to process any emotions that are still heavily linked to your story of herpes: how you got it, who gave it to you, how it has effected your life, and how people may have responded to you negatively. Get out a pen and paper and begin to write out your story. Write down every little bit of detail you can remember: What was the weather like when you were diagnosed? What time*

of year was it? What was going on in your life at the time of diagnosis? The more detail you can bring to your story, the better your results will be. Write down your whole story in a single sitting. Have a box of tissues by your side as you write. Play some really sappy music to evoke all of your emotions!

2. Be in your sadness, and let it flow into your words. Don't edit as you go; just get it all on paper.

3. When you have written the last of your story, arrange a time and place for you to share it with someone you feel comfortable with—maybe your mother, a sister, or a best friend. It is best to ask someone you can be face-to-face with. If this is not possible, you can always share your story in front of a mirror, although this is not the preferred method.

4. Instruct your partner not to respond in any way other than a gentle nod. Do not allow him or her to speak. Turn off all cell phones and rid yourself of any distractions. Get knee to knee and eye to eye. Read your story aloud from beginning to end.

5. During this process, you will probably feel the full weight of your story. Let your feelings fly! Don't hold back!

6. Once you are done with your first read-through, take a deep breath and begin again. Reread your entire story until you can read it without feeling any emotion in your body.

7. This is a continuous process and is not to be interrupted. Do not allow any talking or distractions between your readings.

8. These emotions might be locked deep within your body. Don't be surprised if you begin to laugh at yourself by about the fifth or maybe tenth time you read your story. Don't stop until you reach a place in which your story has no emotional charge. Don't stop until you reach this point. You might take an hour or more to release all of your negative emotions.

9. Once you reach the other side, you can talk to your partner and accept a warm embrace. Be sure to burn your story when you have completed this exercise. You are now ready to have "the Talk" and to move forward in life.

Some people find relief in bodywork that addresses these traumas. The hip area is often a huge depot for these stored emotions. Consider receiving a massage, some Reiki, emotional freedom technique (EFT), chiropractic, or any number of other approaches that are known to work with trauma in the emotional body. This might be the perfect finishing touch to this powerful exercise.

Eliminating Your Fears before Having "the Talk"—An Exercise

What you can't be with controls you.

—UNKNOWN AUTHOR

Illuminating Your Shadows

Have you ever heard the saying "what you resist persists"? This is a popular belief in the world of personal growth and transformation. What you cannot be with, or what it is that you resist, might unveil an aspect of your life we will call your shadow. Your shadow is the part of yourself that you desperately try to hide from others. For most of us, our shadow involves tales of embarrassment, shame, personal weaknesses, and fears. But it is from our shadows that we can gain the most momentum and energy to experience a breakthrough in life. When our shadows are filled with fear, our minds weave stories of worst-case scenarios, and all of our decisions are made from this place. Once we can illuminate our shadows, our medicine for change emerges. This is an exercise that will eliminate your fears around having "the Talk." The things in your head are stronger and harsher than reality.

Let's say you have a fear of snakes. When you even think of them, your hands get sweaty, your heart begins to pound, and you imagine being bitten and dying from a poisonous bite. If this is true, you might never take up gardening, despite the fact that you've always dreamed of tending to a garden. You'll spend your whole life avoiding places that might harbor snakes. This is a pretty big section of the outdoors to avoid! If you won a free trip to Australia, which is known to have lots of snakes, you would never be able to go due to your current relationship to snakes. Forget about your dreams of seeing the Great Barrier Reef!

What if you could move beyond your fear? An entirely new world would open up for you. This might be uncomfortable for you, but the truth is that your chances of encountering a snake are very small. The odds of being bitten are even smaller. A study presented by the University of Florida shows that you are nine times as likely to die from being struck by lightening than from being bitten by a poisonous snakebite! This is a perfect example of a fear commonly blown out of proportion when compared to the actual reality of the threat. When you can be present with things you fear most, they quickly begin to lose their power over you.

Full steam ahead! Overcome your fears and start living your life. Most people who have herpes initially fear that no one will ever love them again. It is not uncommon to fear the worst possible outcome when telling a potential partner. These negative thoughts can resurface if it has been a long time since you last had "the Talk" with a past partner. When your mind is consumed with worst-case scenarios, you seek refuge by pushing away any opportunity for intimacy because of the underlying fear of rejection. FEAR, as Jack Canfield often reminds us, is False Evidence Appearing Real. Now that is worth memorizing!

The following exercise will invite your shadows into the light. It is from this place, and only this place, that your thoughts and your outcomes can be transformed. If you want to attract the perfect mate but you hold the body language of rejection and low self-esteem, you will not be able to attract a confident, healthy mate.

This is an amazing exercise to find grace in your relationship with herpes. Do not be surprised if this exercise elicits some deep feelings. Be gentle with yourself as you work through each scenario.

Also, be sure to quote your "imaginary" lover, mother, father, sister, or brother. These imaginary versions of the people in your life are much harsher with you. All of your thoughts, shadows, and nightmares are concerned with these imaginary people, not the actual people and what they might say.

Write down a sentence that your imaginary lover could say to you that would really hurt your feelings:

Write down a sentence that your imaginary mother could say to you that would really hurt your feelings:

Write down a sentence that your imaginary father could say to you that would really hurt your feelings:

Write down a sentence that your imaginary sister or brother could say to you that would really hurt your feelings:

Write down a sentence that your imaginary friend could say to you that would really hurt your feelings:

Now, rewrite the first sentence, but change it from a "you" statement to an "I" statement, and add the word "sometimes." So, for example, if the cruel thing your imaginary lover said was "You are so promiscuous," then you would write, "I am promiscuous sometimes."

Now slowly read that sentence aloud a few times. Feel it in your body. Try to just be with it. Is it true? Could it be true that you are sometimes that way? Even once? Can you think of a specific time when this was true? Can you accept this in a peaceful way?

Repeat this process with each sentence, attempting only to feel some peace around each one. If the second sentence is "You embarrass me," then you would write and say aloud, "I am embarrassing sometimes." Is it true? Have you ever embarrassed anyone? Are there times when you have not been an embarrassment but rather someone to be proud of?

When you can develop the ability to gracefully sit with any self-concept that frightens you, you will be able to go anywhere and do anything. Once you have worked through your fears with "the Talk," use this exercise for any shadows lurking in the dark, and continue your journey of self-discovery, growth, and healing.

In Parting

I learn by going where I have to go.

—THEODORE ROETHKE

When life presents you with a bowl full of lemons, what do you do? Make lemonade! Surrender to this journey, and know you will come out on the other side, better and stronger than ever. Just as when you have self-respect, others will respect you, when you love yourself, you allow yourself to be fully loved by others. Do you know people who truly honor, value, and respect their unique selves? Do they seem more physically attractive than those who do the exact opposite? I believe it has to do with a level of transparency and authenticity. Think of Oprah Winfrey. We are endlessly drawn to her because she has always remained authentic to her viewers and has never been afraid to show her emotions. Knowing who you are does not mean coming from a place of ego. It is a quiet confidence, speaking with body language rather than verbal language. It is more of the presence of being as opposed to doing. When you can truly embrace all of who you are, and I mean everything, down to your "imperfect" second toe, then you are on a path to greatness and on a path to serve humanity.

Herpes is a blessing in disguise. Be open to receiving these blessings. As children, we often don't know that we are growing until we must buy a new pair of shoes. Our parents notice it, but we might not. Internal growth can be hard to measure, too, and although you are learning and growing, it might take an outside friend or family member to notice. Personal growth occurs most rapidly when we are placed under stress—and yes, a herpes diagnosis is stressful. Just think of it this way: it takes a tremendous amount of heat and pressure to form one of the strongest and most beautiful elements on earth, a diamond. If you are feeling over-whelmed and wobbly, stop, breathe, and regroup. You are a diamond in the rough.

Is it your fault that you contracted the herpes virus? No. But what I am saying is that a "perfect storm" was at play to uncover self-love and radical forgiveness, should you choose to take the lessons on. Maybe this was exactly what you needed to grow as a person. If you allow yourself to receive these gifts, you can then take them into every area of your life and continue your journey of spiritual growth and evolution. Taking full responsibility for everything that transpires in your life is easy when things are going well, and challenging when they aren't. Just as soon as you think you have a grasp of this thing called life, or even your herpes, you'll be thrown a curve ball.

When faced with this philosophical quandary of whether or not you are responsible for everything that happens in your life, it is logical to fall into the questioning of why horrific things exist in this world. Why are there massive amounts of famine, disease, and heartache? Why were you or a loved one infected with herpes? From a macroscopic perspective, the universe is divine and perfect, and there are spiritual laws that lie far beyond a level of consciousness that we might never understand.

Beneath the Pink Tent

It is my vision to use my experience of herpes to bring women together in a sacred space to further explore self-love, health, and well-being. Dating back to biblical times, women used to spend a great deal of time together in women-only environments. For example, when you would enter your moon cycle (menses) or begin labor, you would leave your husband and enter "the red tent," a place where women gathered to support one another. Mothers, grandmothers, friends, sisters, aunts, great grandmothers, and medicine women would gather and support you in connection, celebration, rejuvenation, healing, and spiritual ritual.

Remember what it was like when you were a little girl at a slumber party? What did you talk about? Did you look up at the midnight sky, speaking of fairies, princes, and toads? Did you giggle the night away? Did you talk about boys and your latest crush? Did you play truth-or-dare? Of course you did! Why is it that as we grow up, we spend less and less time with the women we love? You know the magic that occurs when women gather. I invite you to join me in the creation of a new place to dream, ask questions, get inspired, be heard, explore spirituality, embrace health, laugh, sing, and cry. In celebration of the red tent of antiquity, I have created the "pink tent" (www.pinktent.com), a safe place for women to gather and support one another on their healing path to live, love, and thrive. This is a groundbreaking multimedia platform where you can unveil the mask, connect woman to woman, and discover the nurturing you deserve.

You are no longer alone, and it's time you nourish your soul in community. Find out what has worked for other women with herpes, or ask about personal growth and transformation. Once you feel supported, then you can support others. This just might be the perfect platform from which you will fly. Maybe you will begin volunteering your time in a nearby soup kitchen; maybe you will start a nonprofit, quit your job, travel the world, or commit to being a better mother or wife. Whatever it is, know that Pink Tent will support you in all of your endeavors toward healthy living.

Live. Love. Thrive.

Dr. Kelly

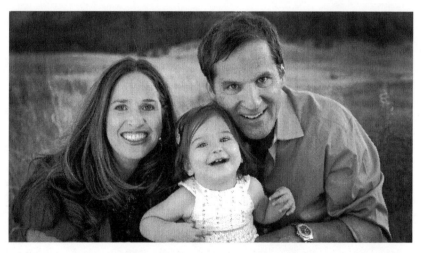

Richard, Madeline and Me

Exercises and Meditations

Below is a compilation of some of my favorite meditations and exercises for healing and rebalancing the body, mind, and soul. Although there are several exercises sprinkled throughout the text, this section is meant to be a grab-and-go section. Being an active participant in your healing journey is paramount. If you take the time to do these exercises, you will learn how to live a more vibrant, heart-centered life while learning how to keep your herpes symptoms at bay.

Take just one exercise at a time and incorporate it into your life. In general, I recommend choosing one meditation or exercise and working with it for a week or so. This is your journey, so follow your intuition on your healing path.

My PINK Diary Is Cool!

I began journaling when I was in junior high. Writing down all of my thoughts and feelings was my secret garden. It is amazing how this sacred space has carried me into adulthood and now motherhood. Over the years, my journal has been a place that I can go to and share my wildest dreams and most private thoughts. It is my personal pink tent where my magic wand, tiara, and fairies still greet me.

Journals have the power to create a sacred space of inspiration and personal growth. Whenever one journal ends, a new one begins. I love shopping for a new journal. Will it be sparkly, artistic, or filled with poems and quotes?

Go out and purchase a journal specifically to document your healing process. Write in it every day. My journal entries totally shifted after I read Julia Campbell's book *The Artist's Way*. Don't let the title intimidate you, for everyone is an artist in his or her own right. Her book taught me the concept of writing during the morning, unedited and free-flowing. When I began this process, I realized how judgmental I was being of my own thoughts. Use this method to get the words and feelings outside of your head and onto the paper. No one will ever read these entries except for you.

When I decided to write this book, I pulled out my old journals and was able to discover how my emotional relationship to herpes healed over the years. I realized that over time, I was able identify what triggered emotional states that then triggered outbreaks.

Don't feel like you have to write about herpes every day. Just write down what is on your mind. In addition to this fluid form of writing, I want you to write down some facts. Follow the self-care plan. Set short-term and long-term goals. Chart your outbreaks, your triggers, your supplements, your story sharing, and any other "facts" that will help you better understand yourself and your herpes. No two journeys will be the same. Learn what your body is teaching you in this journey of self-discovery and relationships. Be your own healer.

Create a sticker program with colorful hearts, smiley faces, and stars. We are all still children at heart, and we respond to rewards and the tracking of success. Set a goal in regards to the above recommendations, and each day you reach your goal, you get a sticker. For the daily practices, start small. It is next to impossible to make changes if you try to use an all-or-nothing approach. Remember, it is more important to start in the right direction than to go on and off this program totally. Once you get to the point that you are outbreak free for three or more months, then, and only then, consider reintroducing possible triggers, one at a time.

Meditation Made Simple

Take a minimum of fifteen minutes a day to practice meditation. The best time to meditate is first thing in the morning and right before bedtime. This is when your mind is the most open to receive the blessings of meditation. To begin, focus on your breath. When your mind wanders, come back to your breath. When a thought arises, imagine a chalkboard in front of you. Write the name of the thought, and then take a large eraser and erase the thought from the board. Then, sink back into your breath. This is a great practice to clear the clutter from your monkey mind and to discover peace and clarity in your day-to-day life. If you don't "have time," create time by waking up fifteen minutes earlier than you normally would. Set an alarm clock if you need to. Meditation will sprinkle a bit of fairy dust in your life, allowing for miracles in mind, body, and spirit to be called forth.

Rejuvenating Meditation

It is not uncommon to feel totally exhausted during viral outbreaks. Use the following meditation as a tool to give your body the down time that it needs. I have found that even fifteen minutes of this meditation can rejuvenate the body as if you had an hour or more of deep sleep.

Close your eyes and begin to notice the rising ebb and flow of your breath cycles. Bring your attention to a point between your eyes, in the middle of your brain, also known as the third eye or the seat of consciousness. This is the site where the pineal gland resides. The pineal gland is an endocrine gland about the size of a pea, and it is very important for regulating sleep cycles.

Rest your hands, palms up, on your legs. While keeping your spine straight, surrender to the weight of gravity. Imagine that in your hands you are holding the head of a sleeping baby. Feel into the gentleness, vibrancy, and love of the infant. Feel the weight of its head in your hands. Imagine that this baby is you. Return to your innocence and trust. Allow your love to outpour through your hands. Feel the buzz of this precious life. Continue breathing in and out slowly through your nose. When you feel complete, give thanks for this moment of silence.

Take a few more deep breaths and slowly open your eyes. Give yourself time to reenter the world around you.

Building Self-Confidence

I saw the angel in the marble and carved until I set him free.

—MICHELANGELO

Repeat after me: "I am amazing." Again, one more time with gusto, "I am amazing." Say this over and over again until you feel a bit giddy. There is no one else in the world like you. You are a beautiful and unique individual. You are a goddess, and *everything* about you is perfect!

Take a moment and think of other challenges you have had in your life and how you overcame them. Make a list of the attributes you must have had in place to overcome these obstacles.

Now, add to the list:

Three Things You LOVE about Yourself
1.
2.
3.

Three Things You LOVE about Your Body
1.
2.
3.

Three Things You LOVE about Your Mind
1.
2.
3.

Three Things You LOVE about Your Spirit
1.
2.
3.

Write this on a different piece of paper and place it in an area of your home where you can see it daily. Get in touch with your inner angel, who is magnificent beyond measure, and set her free to expect miracles in your life.

Raising the Roof of Self-Esteem

In the world of duality, cold cannot exist without hot, up without down, and happiness without sadness. Zen philosophy teaches of the power that exists in neutrality, a still point of sorts.

When we are diagnosed with herpes, we experience several negative emotions and feelings about ourselves, which are detrimental to our self-esteem and our ability to heal. When we are able to step into our greatest fears and acknowledge our self-deprecating self-talk and self-concept, we can embrace the darkness and move forward. This exercise moves you out of your head and into you body. This is somatic healing at its best!

In order to do this exercise, it is best to be in a quiet place with no distractions. All you need is a piece of paper and a pen. First, fold your paper in half and create two columns. In the first column, write down a list of all of the negative things you tell yourself in regards to herpes and how it might affect your life. It is extremely powerful when you can begin each statement with "I am." Do not use the word "not" in any of these statements, for it tends to confuse your subconscious mind. Take the time to think of *everything* that you have been thinking and telling yourself since your diagnosis. Stop only after you can no longer think of any other negative thoughts.

A list of possible thoughts might include:

I am helpless.
I am unlovable.
I am angry.
I am shameful.

In the second column, write the direct opposite (positive versus negative) of the original thought. For example:

I am empowered.
I am totally lovable.

I am peaceful and happy.
I am proud.

Wherever you are, pick three places you could stand in a room to represent three points of a triangle, positions A, B, and C. Ideally, positions A, B, and C are some distance across the room from one another. First, stand in position A and review your first thought. Speak this thought out loud, and feel into all of the feelings associated with this thought. Try to identify where in your body this feeling resides. Is it in your heart, your head, or some exotic place like your knee? Feel into this thought and allow the feelings to increase. Continue to speak the thought until it no longer amplifies a response or feeling in your body.

Now, move to position B in the room, which represents the thoughts from the second column. Speak the first thought out loud several times. Think of things that would "prove" this to be true. Think of experiences you have had that embrace the positive thought. Where do you feel these feelings when you think about them? In the beginning, you might have a challenging time embodying these emotions, but I guarantee they exist beneath all of those negative emotions. Maybe you can only feel empowered at the tip of your pinky finger, but it is there, somewhere in a memory. Allow these feelings to expand in your body.

Stand in position C, a triad point between position A and B. This is the still point, the place where neither opposite exists. It is where a pendulum stops and no longer wavers. Begin by stepping into position A and repeating statement number one. Feel into it and then move onto position B. Speak that statement again. Move back to position C and see if you can hold both thoughts at the same time. If it is easier, imagine the thought from position A resides in your right hand and the thought from position B resides in your left hand. Now hold both thoughts at the same time.

Some people find it useful to continue to walk to the different positions until they are truly able to find the still point, C, in their body. Most people experience the still point as a relief. Their mind begins to quiet, and a level of peace overcomes them. It is from this powerful place of neutrality that the healing of opposites begins to take place.

We are all of these things that we think of at some point in time. When we can embrace and honor our feelings, our mind can begin to calm down, and we can begin to experience our true nature, our higher self, which has no name. It is the nameless.

Sushi-Size Your Day

I *love* sushi. The little bites fill me with delight. The colors, presentation, and refreshing feeling I have after I have eaten it all contribute to the experience. I think it is the simplicity of the Zen presentation and attention to detail that lure me in. When life gets overwhelming or out of sync, I remember to take the time to sushi-size my day.

Overwhelm and negative thoughts and feelings are all things we can choose to live with…or to live without. Begin your day with sushi-sized intentions. Clearly decide how you want your morning to look, rather than thinking of *everything* you must accomplish in the day. If you are feeling negative or sad, think of just one thing you are grateful for or one thing that makes you happy.

It is much easier to manage your life when you can consciously intend it, bit by bit or bite by bite. I have found this exercise to be extremely powerful in my life. All you have to do is to stop yourself, take a deep breath, and *decide* what the next, say, fifteen minutes could look like, and begin to move in that direction. Let's say that you are late to work and are hitting every stop sign, red light, and accident. Take a minute and sushi-size or compartmentalize the experience. Think of open lanes, green lights, and gratitude. While you're at it, intend the perfect parking space as you roll into work. The exercise is as simple as that!

For some, this positive intention setting needs to be practiced on an hourly basis. Hours turn into days and then weeks. Bringing presence to everything you do will become a habit that only needs occasional reminders. It is amazing how, with time, your sushi-sizing will leave you feeling light upon the earth with peace in your heart.

Accessing Your Inner Guru

Your inner guru is always with you, guiding you in life whether you listen to her or not. Every day you are faced with challenges and problems that you need to work through. It can be exhausting being in a place of indecision while you weigh out every permutation of all of your possible outcomes.

If I shared with you a powerful exercise you could use for nearly any obstacle found in your life, would you use it? I hope so. Accessing your inner guru is much easier when you can take one step outside of your-self. A diagnosis of herpes can lead you to ask many internal questions. *What remedy should I try first, when should I have "the Talk," should I attempt to go off my antiviral prescription, should I talk to the person I think gave me herpes, should I try a cleanse, how do I break my addiction to chocolate?* These are just a few of the internal debates you might be having with yourself. Whenever a question like this arises, here is what you can do to gain clarity.

Ideally, you should do this exercise with a friend, but you can also do it solo by writing out the question and response. If you choose to do this exercise with a friend, here is how you would do it. Tell your friend all about your problem. Then, have him or her say:

"I have an amazing friend (you) who has this problem:" (At this point, have your friend repeat to you what your problem is.)

Then, have your friend ask you, "What advice do you have for my friend?"

You will be surprised what occurs to you when you are hearing someone else tell your story. I have found that people are much more compassionate and clear when they are listening to a problem they want to help their friend solve. If you do not have a partner to share with, simply write this out for yourself:

I have an amazing friend who has this problem:

What advice do I have for this person?. (Take the perspective of giving advice to a good friend.)

Thank you. That is wonderful advice!

A List of De-stressors

In keeping with the theme of nurturing and nourishing yourself during this time, I encourage you to make a list of things that de-stress you. I have always had a list like this in the back of my journals. The key here is to ask yourself, "What brings me out of fear and into love?" In other words, what calms your mind, opens your heart, and brings you peace and love?

Every time I discover something new, I add it to my list. Here's a list of my favorite gentle things to de-stress:

- doing yoga
- meditation
- receiving massage or other bodywork
- taking a long, candlelit bath
- going to a bookstore and buying a new book
- calling someone I love
- cuddling with my husband, baby, and kitty
- writing random thank-you notes
- watching a romantic comedy
- watching the sun set
- drinking vanilla rooibos tea
- walking a labyrinth
- going for a mindful hike
- creating a fabulous meal
- photographing my baby

Feel free to steal any one of my ideas. While you wrap yourself in self-love, consider yourself hugged by me. If I could be right there with you, I would. I would remind you of your gifts and the light that you are here to shine upon the world.

Daily Dose

Before I met Richard, I was the type of woman you would find in the self-help and spirituality sections of the Boulder Bookstore on a Saturday afternoon. For a while I was a personal-growth and self-help junkie. I attended workshops all around the nation, read books, and spoke with friends, searching for the magic behind manifestation. My life began to mirror those I read about. As my commitment to my dreams grew stronger, uncanny synchronism became a part of my everyday life.

Each night before I went to bed, I read through a series of about ten affirmations that I had written out in colorful markers on index cards. The last thing my eyes saw before I went to bed was my dream board, a collection of images and words that captured my dreams. I began living into a world I was creating. I awoke each morning to meditate and run or hike on the trails of Boulder. As the sun rose over the mountaintops, my eyes gazed across the endless miles of flatlands that extended from the foothills to the fields in Kansas. I purposely left my tunes at home so that I could connect to the earth and to my internal biorhythms. All I could hear was the pounding of my heart, the dirt trail beneath my feet, and the bellowing of my lungs.

As my body was running like a fluid machine across the rocky terrain, my mind would finally release. I began each run with my top ten things of the day that I was grateful for. I would then move into envisioning the man of my dreams. How I would feel when I was with him? What would he smell like? What would we do together? I envisioned skiing, eating a candlelit dinner, and laughing with him. I even remember thinking what it would be like to cuddle with him under the covers on a cold winter day. I got as vivid as I could.

After creating these images in my mind, I would verbally speak my affirmations. My affirmations were short and sweet and repeated several times between a runner's pant. No two morning runs were exactly the same, but the overall feeling of my life expanding into a whole new world of possibilities felt amazing. This dedication to finding my soul mate opened me up to him coming into my life. It was like doing mental repetitions in the gym. Did you know that the mind has a tough time distinguishing between the "real-life imagery" you create and the "reality" that you live? Use this to your advantage.

Dr. Kelly's Guide to Healing Modalities

Healing is a journey and not a destination. At this point, it should come as no surprise that I believe that healing modalities should be implemented into your life now, whether you have symptoms or not. The mere act of living places a great deal of stress on your body, and the day-to-day, year-to-year stresses will eventually catch up to you. Implementing some healing modalities into your self-care plan will lead you to greater states of health and well-being.

Many people wait until they have symptoms to get help. This approach is akin to never doing maintenance on your car until it breaks down. Managing herpes is no different than putting gas in your tank, rotating your tires, and changing out the oil in your car.

If you can view your body as a well-oiled machine, making a commitment to use these healing modalities will keep your body in tiptop shape. Prevention will keep your herpes at bay. If you want to live a vibrant, healthy life, reach in and reach out. We were never meant to take this journey alone!

Acupuncture: Originated in China over five thousand years ago, acupuncture is based on the belief that the balance of vital life energy, present in all living organisms, determines health. Acupuncture theory is based on twelve major energy pathways, called meridians, which are linked to specific internal organs and organ systems. Needles are inserted into acupoints (just under the skin) that help rebalance the flow of energy in specific organ systems, alleviating pain and restoring health.

Applied Kinesiology: This method is used to identify and treat a vast variety of health problems. It is based on the belief that there is a close relationship between a muscle dysfunction and a related organ or gland dysfunction, causing a specific health problem. Various techniques are then applied in order to strengthen the muscles involved with the dysfunction, thus restoring health.

Aromatherapy: A unique aspect of herbal medicine, aromatherapy utilizes the medicinal properties found in the essential oils of various aromatic plants. Oils are extracted from flowers, branches, leaves, and roots. The small molecular size of oils makes them a unique healing agent because they can easily be absorbed through bodily tissues. These oils are used in a variety of healing applications to rebalance the mind, body, and soul. The oils have antimicrobial, antiviral, and antifungal properties. Oils are used topically, inhaled, and diffused into the air. Aromatherapy oils such as Melissa, olive leaf, tea tree oil, and lavender are a few oils that have shown to be effective against the herpes virus.

Ayurvedic Medicine: This comprehensive system of medicine combines natural therapies with a personalized approach to the treatment of disease. It places parallel emphasis on mind, body, and spirit and strives to restore harmony within an individual. Each body is characterized by its metabolic type or its constitution, namely Vata, Pitta, and Kapha. When these are in balance, the body is in balance, and health is restored. An Ayurvedic doctor determines the constitution of an individual and then creates a healing regimen that includes dietary changes, exercise, yoga, meditation, massage, and herbal tonics.

Biofeedback Training: This somatic technique teaches how to shift and control the body's vital functions using an electronic device. This method of learning how to consciously regulate a normally unconscious bodily function, such as heart rate and blood pressure, helps to enhance overall health. This is an excellent method of choice for those who are hypervigilant, stressed, and anxious.

Bodywork: This form of mind-body medicine includes a wide range of techniques including deep- and soft-tissue massage, sports massage, Reiki, foot reflexology, Qigong, chiropractic, breath work, and energy medicine to realign the body, correct postural imbalances, and produce a heightened state of body awareness. These differing approaches de-stress the nervous system and allow the body to return to health. Many ailments are healed through bodywork.

Chiropractic: Chiropractic is a natural, drug-free, and surgery-free approach to heath. At its core, chiropractic focuses on the integrity of the nervous system, the body's master system, to determine imbalances within the body. Chiropractors detect and correct misalignments of the spine, alleviating pain and enhancing health. It has become the second-largest leading health-care field in the world with effectiveness in treating headaches, back problems, and many other medical conditions. If you have genital herpes and have had trauma or surgery to your spine, especially your low back and pelvis, you might consider using the care of a chiropractor. They can remove nerve interference in your pelvis that might be contributing to your genital outbreaks. My favorite approach to chiropractic, outside of Flowtrition, is Network Spinal Analysis. It is a very gentle approach to chiropractic and extremely powerful in its ability to release old stress and trauma held within the body.

Colon Therapy: This therapy promotes a healthy and functional colon that can ease a variety of problems most commonly including allergies, Candida, headaches, weight gain, and fatigue. If you suffer from constipation, dehydration, or you are living in America, your colon is backed up with toxins. What goes in should come out, but too often it doesn't! Colon therapy irrigates and detoxifies the lower intestine with water. This area of the colon cannot be reached with enemas. Once the colon is flushed of old waste, it can then be repopulated with healthy probiotics or gut flora. This helps to restore balance in the body chemistry and allows the body to restore proper tissue and organ functions.

Craniosacral Therapy: In this therapy typically used by osteopaths, naturopaths, and chiropractors, the practitioner uses his/her hands to assess the motion of the craniosacral system (the head and spinal systems). Improper movement of the bones of the skull has been linked to a wide variety of illnesses and diseases from ear infections to cerebral palsy. The goal of the treatment is to restore the proper flow of CSF (cerebral spinal fluid) in the body and to realign any misaligned bones in the system. This leads to an overall increase in health of the nervous system and helps to restore balance in the system.

Cryotherapy: Cryotherapy uses cold temperatures locally or environmentally to heal the body. You are probably familiar with the use of ice on boo-boos, but did you know that ice packs can be very beneficial for someone who is suffering from a herpes outbreak? Placing an ice pack or frozen bag of veggies on your herpes sores can help to decrease the pain and the local metabolism and enzymatic activity of those crazy, replicating herpes cells. The cold temperatures will also decrease swelling and inflammation, the cornerstones of pain. Initially, the application of cold will cause the blood supply in the area to constrict, followed by reflexive vasodilation or warming of the area after the ice is removed. This rush of new blood to the area essentially flushes out the old toxins and dead cells as it also replenishes the area with new nutrients and cells for healing.

Detoxification Therapy: This helps remove chemicals and pollutants within the body and restore health by cleansing or neutralizing the liver, kidneys, urine, and feces. We now carry an obscene amount of toxins in our body, ranging from industrial chemicals to food additives, heavy metals, pesticides, and residues from pharmaceutical drugs. This causes our immune system to break down and disease to set in. Detoxification therapy utilizes water or juice fasts, along with a specialized diet, to aid the body in releasing the toxins and restoring health. Once the toxins are removed, the tissues and cells are then able to restore and rejuvenate themselves and return to a heightened level of healing capacity. This therapy has been shown to be effective in the treatment of obesity, arthritis, cancer, diabetes, and overall bodily function.

Diet: A diet contributes to an incredibly large portion to how our body and brain function. A diet high in white flower, red meat, refined starches, and additives and pesticides contributes to heart disease, stroke, and cancer. Preservatives, antibiotics, and hormones within dairy and animal products, as well as chemicals and pesticides within some of our food, play a major part in birth defects, decreased immune function, cancer, destruction of nerve tissue, and food allergies. A whole-foods diet, a foundation of mostly cooked plants and some meat, is a healthy diet. Raw foods and juice, fermented foods, and garlic, ginger, and yeasts provide great additions to your list of healthy foods.

EMDR (Eye Movement Desensitization and Reprocessing): This is a form of psychotherapy that is an information-processing therapy. It is based on the belief that past experiences directly effect and trigger current pathologies. In this therapy, past experiences are addressed in order to produce more adaptive behaviors and mental health for the future. During a process called dual stimulation, a client might recall a past event while using eye movements, taps, or tones. While attending to these external stimuli, the client is then asked to recall past memories, triggers, or anticipated future experiences. While doing this process, clients report new insights, associations, and memories. This technique can be very powerful for those with herpes, helping them remove their emotional triggers to herpes.

Energy Medicine: By using a variation of diagnostic screening devices to measure the variations of electromagnetic frequencies produced by the body, it is possible to detect imbalances that may cause illness and future disease. Once an imbalance is identified, holistic therapies and treatment devices are used in order to rebalance the energy levels. This therapy is based on acupuncture's meridian system, where different organs are associated with specific meridian points. There are many types of energy medicine, such as the electroacupuncture biofeedback devices, which have been known to detect almost all known diseases, toxicity, and food allergies.

Environmental Medicine: This discipline explores the role of dietary and environmental allergens in relationship to illness and health. Specific foods, molds, chemicals, and dust can contribute to anything from common colds to depression. Through diet, skin, and thyroid-function tests, it is possible to understand what needs to be eliminated from the surrounding environment in order to improve health. For example, a patient with severe rheumatoid arthritis might begin to eliminate certain allergy-producing foods, allowing the body to heal and the symptoms of arthritis to subside.

Enzyme Therapy: This therapy uses plants and foods to restore digestive-related health problems. The ability to properly digest and absorb nutrients in foods is essential to good health. Vitamins, minerals, and hormones depend on enzymes to function properly. Many of the digestive enzymes are made in the pancreas, and their role in metabolism is to break down food and help with the absorption of nutrients into the blood. These enzymes are also responsible for building new cells and repairing damaged ones in the blood, tissues, and organs. Many chronic illnesses, including multiple sclerosis, cancer, inflammation, autoimmune disorders, and viral diseases, are being treated successfully with the addition of these enzymes to the diet.

Fasting: This cost-effective therapy aids a variety of symptoms. Fasting allows the body to rid itself of toxins and stimulate healing, because energy is no longer being consumed for digestion. There are water and juice fasts (essentially a restricted diet) that release toxins and eliminate waste from the body. While fasting can be beneficial, it is not for everyone. Those with eating disorders, epilepsy, terminal illness, etc., should not fast except under professional supervision. Please consult with your doctor to learn more.

Flower Remedies: The source of these remedies? You guessed it, flowers! These remedies directly impact our emotional state in order to expedite physiological and psychological well-being. Flower remedies, with incredible effectiveness, remove emotional barriers to health and recovery. These remedies are based on Dr. Bach's (founder of Bach Flower Remedies) theory that emotional unhappiness and illness are directly related to physical illness. Searching for a holistic approach to healing, Dr. Bach focused on flowers and discovered thirty-eight flowering plants and trees that were able to soothe psychological and emotional states that heavily influenced physical illness. Each remedy is said to trigger the body into its own internal healing process. The flower remedy does not directly treat a physical ailment. However, it does treat a psychological or emotional state contributing to the physical disease. For example, sunflower coincides with self-worth, while fuchsia coincides with the repression of deep-seated emotions.

Guided Imagery: This therapy utilizes the imagination to reduce stress and stimulate the immune system. It can be used to help create insight into a past event or to heal a current health condition. The body is constantly reacting to imagery or thoughts, creating physical symptoms. Although thoughts exist in the mind, the body reacts to them. Imagery is often used to stimulate healing within the body and can assist in defining emotions, behaviors, and attitudes that might be involved in creating illnesses in the body. It is used for recovery from cancer, depression, and chronic inflammatory disease.

Herbal Medicine: Herbal (herb) medicine is one of if not the most ancient form of medicine known. From South America to Northern Africa to the tops of Everest to Southeast Asia, communities around the world still utilize some form of herbal medicine in their healing process. Most pharmaceuticals used today are derived from trees, herbs, and shrubs or synthesized to mimic a medicinal plant compound. Spices, herbs, fruit, bark, seed, step, and root are all used in herbal medicine. Herbs can treat chronic illness, rheumatic and arthritic conditions, allergies, and respiratory issues; or they can be used to soothe a cut or help mend a broken bone. The list is endless. Whether in a tea, tablet, or capsule form, in an extract, tincture, oil, balm, or salve, there are more than half a dozen ways to implement herbal medicine into your daily diet for prevention or treatment. See the "Healing Remedies" section on page 156 to learn more about how herbs can help you to effectively manage your herpes.

Homeopathy: This nontoxic system of medicine used worldwide is incredibly effective in treating chronic illness that does not respond to conventional medicine. Homeopathic medicine is derived from plants, animals, and minerals, and usually presented in a diluted carrier like a tablet or a liquid. German physician Samuel Hahneman developed homeopathy at the end of the eighteenth century. Dr. Hahneman revolutionized barbaric methods of health care at the time and sought out cures from the natural environment. In this practice and philosophy, like cures like. For instance, Dr. Hahneman once ingested Peruvian bark (known to cure malaria) daily and began to experience symptoms of malaria. Once he discontinued use of this bark, his symptoms diminished. He then theorized that if the bark created the symptoms of the disease in a healthy being, then it could cure the same disease in a person suffering from it. He then discovered that small doses of the bark could stimulate healing in a person suffering from malaria. His system of "like cures like" is the foundation of every homeopathic remedy. It's fascinating really—do your research on this brilliant man! The most common homeopathic remedies used to treat herpes are Rhus-tox, Mezereum, and Ranunculus.

Hypnotherapy: Through a trance-like state, it is possible to access the subconscious brain in order to change behavior so that health conditions (mental disorders, fear, phobias, depression, and physical pain) can be relieved. Through verbal communication, the hypnotherapist slowly induces the patient into deep states of relaxation and essentially manipulates the patient into thinking he or she is healthy, healing, or healed from a specific ailment. There is an astonishingly high success rate with herpes.

Juice Therapy: This therapy uses the juicing of fresh vegetables, fruits, and herbs for healing. Juicing is a technique that removes the pulp and extracts the nutrients. The removal of the pulp allows the body to more easily digest the nutrients. Juicing is a great way to flush your body with nutrients and to remove toxic substances. It has also been used to fight disease, improve immunity, encourage weight loss, improve mental health, and reduce the risk of several chronic conditions. I personally use juicing for everyday nutrition and as a means to detoxify the body.

Low-Level Laser Therapy (LLLT): This form of therapy has been growing in popularity in recent years in the field of alternative medicine.

LLLT uses a cold laser to therapeutically treat an area of the body without injuring or damaging the cell. This form of light therapy provides energy in the form of nonthermal photons of light. The light then stimulates the production of collagen, ATP, and enzymes, which are all essential for cellular repair of damaged tissue. LLLT is also known to strengthen the immune system, decrease pain, and decrease inflammation. There have been reports of people with herpes responding positively to the treatment.

Meditation: Meditation is a technique to quiet the mind and attain heightened levels of awareness and feelings of well-being. Some people also use meditation as a form of prayer. Although this technique has been used since antiquity, it is practiced in numerous forms.

Naturopathic Medicine: This is a form of alternative medicine that has its roots in theories of vitalism, which states that the body is controlled by a vital energy that controls all bodily processes including metabolism, growth, reproduction, and adaptation. This form of medicine is holistic in nature, and it is principled in the belief that the body has an innate ability to heal itself. As a result, naturopaths seek to resolve imbalances in the body with the least amount of intervention. Naturopathic doctors, NDs, use diet, exercise, lifestyle changes, and natural therapies to support their patients in accessing their natural healing intelligence. The term "naturopathy" is translated from the Greek and Latin root "nature disease."

Narrative Therapy: This is a form of psychotherapy that uses narrative as a form of healing. This practice was developed by the ideas and practices of Michael White, David Epston, and other practitioners. The role of narrative therapy is to place clients at the center of their healing journey. It is clients, not therapists, who are thought to have inherent competencies, beliefs, values, skills, and commitments that will assist them in changing their relationships with the problems in their lives. A willingness and curiosity to ask questions to answers they might not know is a cornerstone of the work. A great place to start a narrative therapy journey without a personal therapist is www.pinktent.com. You might find that sharing your story here is cathartic in this safe, supportive environment of other women with herpes.

Nutritional Supplements: If you think you can get all of your nutrients from food, you are delusional! Maybe your grandparents were able to eat an apple a day to keep the doctors away, but we do not have that luxury. We would have to eat ten apples a day to get the same nutritional value. Most nutrients do come from food, but our fruits and veggies are being grown in depleted soils. If the plants are not getting the nutrients from the soil, then by a trickle-down effect, we are not getting our nutrients from the plants. We are also living in a world that is filled with toxins. Combine toxins, stress, and poor nutrition, and you have the perfect ingredients for sickness. With herpes, you must rebuild your immunity, and supplementing is part of the journey. Nutritional supplementation is a means for you to get the nutrients you need. This does not substitute a good diet. Eat more greens *and* get your supplements on!

Qigong: This is a healing and martial art form from ancient China. It uses breathing exercises, movements, and meditation to strengthen and circulate the life energy or qi in the body. Qigong practice is known to produce a peaceful state of mind and to build vitality, immunity, and overall health.

Raindrop Technique Therapy: This is a healing technique that is trademarked by the essential-oil company Young Living. It uses a combination of reflexology, massage, and essential oils to bring the body into electrical and structural alignment. According to Gary Young, the founder of Young Living, the oils are able to kill off viruses, bacteria, and fungal infections found deep within the body. Aromatic oils are applied along the spine. This application helps to align the energy centers of the body and to release old energetic blocks without the use of any hard pressure. I have found this technique to be extremely relaxing and centering.

Reiki: This is a form of energetic medicine that was developed in 1922 by Japanese Buddhist Mikao Usui. This laying-on-of-hands therapy is used as a healing modality for stress reduction and relaxation. It is based on the belief that there is a life energy that moves through the body, and when this life energy is diminished or blocked, it produces stress or illness. Reiki energy is spiritual in nature, although it is not considered a religion. This sometimes-miraculous healing energy is passed down from the Reiki master to the student through a process called an attunement.

Reflexology: This is a non-invasive complementary practice that uses reflex maps and points found on the feet, hands and outer ear. Pressure is applied to these points in order to activate the healing of specific areas of the body. Reflexology is easy to learn and implement into any healing regimen.

Watsu (Water Shiatsu): Watsu is a healing modality that has its roots in Zen Shiatsu. This technique was born in 1980 after Harold Dull began floating people in water as he applied the principles of Zen Shiatsu he had learned in Japan. Watsu is practiced in a heated pool wherein the practitioner gently stretches, rolls, and twists various parts of a client's body. The warm water, womblike in nature, provides the perfect medium to create deep states of waking relaxation. Watsu is an excellent analgesic, stress reducer, and immune builder. Most people who receive Watsu also report a greater sense of connection as a result of floating in another's arms during a session.

Yoga: This is a physical, mental, and spiritual discipline that has its roots in ancient India. In Sanskrit, yoga literally means to "yoke" or "union" mind, body, and soul. The goal of yoga is to attain spiritual insight, tranquility, and union with creation. Yoga comes in many forms and styles. In the West, the word is often interchanged with the physical practice of asanas, or poses. Asanas are only one of eight "limbs" in yoga. Yoga is an excellent practice to quiet the mind, detox and strengthen the body, rebuild the immune system, and prepare the body to heal. I highly recommend it to all who suffer from herpes.

APPENDIX C

Additional Resources

Recommended Books

The Artist's Way by Julia Cameron

The Biology of Belief: Unleashing the Power of Consciousness, Matter, and Miracles by Bruce H. Lipton

Birthing fromWithin: An Extra-Ordinairy Guide to Childbirth Preparation by Pam England and Rob Horowitz

A Course in Miracles by Dr. Helen Schucman

Dear Lover: A Woman's Guide to Men, Sex, and Love's Deepest Bliss by David Deida

Ina May's Guide to Childbirth by Ina May Gaskin

Power Vs. Force: The Hidden Determinants of Human Behavior by David R. Hawkins

There's a Spiritual Solution to Every Problem by Wayne W. Dyer

The Twelve Healers and Other Remedies by Edward Bach

You Can HealYour Life by Louise Hay

Movies

The Business of Being Born

The Cove

Let's Talk about Sex
The Secret
You Can Heal Your Life: The Movie

Web Sites

www.antennasearch.com
www.ashastd.org
www.blessedherbs.com
www.cdc.gov
www.drlwilson.com
www.drmercola.com
www.flowtrition.com
www.internationalmidwives.org
www.lauricidin.com
www.pinktent.com
www.positivesingles.com
www.talkaboutherpes.com

Products/Companies

Analytic Research Labs: hair analysis
Bare Minerals: natural makeup
Bioglide/Divine 9: personal lubricant with carrageenan
Bio Pro: EMF protection
Blessed Herbs: colon cleanse
Dermalogica: aluminum-free deodorant
Gum-omile: oral herpes
Lauricidin: antiviral
Life Force International: wellness products
Nutronix: colloidal silver gel
Toms of Maine fluoride-free toothpaste and natural products
Vita-Myr: mouthwash
Young Living Essential Oils

Inspirational Leaders in Healing, Spirituality and Personal Growth

—a special thanks for their work

Jack Canfield

Deepak Chopra, MD

Wayne Dyer

Donald Epstein, DC

Debbie Ford

Louise Hay

Gay and Katie Hendricks

Jerry and Ester Hicks

Bruce Lipton, PhD

Joseph Mercola, MD

Christine Northrup, MD

Tony Robins

Doreen Virtue

Marianne Williamson

Lawrence Wilson, MD

Lance Wright, DC

References

Alternative Medicine: The Definitive Guide. The Burton Goldberg Group. Future Medicine Publishing, Inc., 1994.

Ebel, Charles, and Anna Wald, MD, MPH. *Managing Herpes: Living and Loving with HSV*. American Health Association, Inc., 2007.

Picozzi, Michele. *Controlling Herpes Naturally: A Practical Guide to Treatment and Prevention*. Southpaw Press, 2006.

Sacks, Stephen L., MD. *The Truth about Herpes*. Gordon Soules Book Publishers Ltd., 1997.

Scipio, Christopher. *Making Peace with Herpes: A Holistic Guide to Overcoming the Stigma and Freeing Yourself from Outbreaks*. Green Sun Press, 2006.

Warren, Terri, RN, NP. *The Good News about the Bad News—Herpes: Everything You Need to Know*. New Harbinger Publication, 2009.

Index

A Course In Miracles, 45, 211

Affirmations, 38, 57, 60-63, 78, 166, 198

Alternative medicine, 22, 30-34, 36, 48, 156

Aluminum 126, 128, 133, 212

Antibodies, 98, 101, 106, 115

Antivirals, 92, 105, 120

  Acyclovir, 92, 119

  Valtrex, 32-33, 105

Arginine. See Triggers.

Asymptomatic shedding, 32, 103-106, 173, 175

Autoinoculation. See Transmission

Baby. See Herpes-Neonatal

Breast cancer, 128, 153-154

Breast-feeding, 111, 115, 117, 156

Centers for Disease Control and Prevention, 85, 99, 113, 160, 180, 212

Chakra, 50, 71-78, 139, 151-152, 152

Chickenpox. See Herpes.

Childbirth. See Pregnancy and delivery

Clean fifteen, 140-142

Cleanse (Detox), 29, 71, 77, 87, 95-96, 98, 103-107, 112, 124, 137, 152-158, 162, 196

Codex alimentarius, 35

Cold sores. See Herpes.

Condoms, 90, 103-104, 138

Copper toxicitiy, 127, 152-153

Copper/Zinc imbalance, 126-12. See also Zinc.

Cosmetics, 127-128, 133, 138

Cytomegalovirus, See Herpes

Dental dams, 104

Dermatome, 94-95

Deodorants. See Toxicities.

Detox. See Cleanse.

Diagnosis, 2, 23-24, 47, 50, 85, 88-89, 92, 99-100, 102

Diet, 124-126, 131, 134-156

Dirty dozen, 141, 145

Discordant couples, 105
Dreams, 19, 65, 68, 71, 198

Environmental Working Group, 124, 141

FDA, 34-36
Fear of rejection, 173, 184
Fertility, 71, 110, 116
First herpes outbreak, 18-20, 93, 97, 120
Food. See Diet and Toxicities.
Flow period, 41-44
Flowtrition, 24, 201, 212
Forgiveness, 45-52, 57-58, 61, 152, 186

Genital herpes. See Herpes.
Gladitorum. See Herpes.
Grief, 20, 39-44

Hair mineral analysis, 124-126
Healing crisis, 26-27, 150-151
Healing modalities, 199-209
    Acupuncture, 112, 200, 203
    Aromatherapy, 200
    Applied kinesiology, 200
    Ayurvedic medicine, 200
    Biofeedback training, 201, 201
    Bodywork, 150, 183, 197, 201
    Chelation therapy, 126
    Chinese medicine, 110, 113, 157, 164
    Chiropractic, 23-25, 48, 165, 183, 201
    Colon therapy, 201
    Craniosacral therapy, 153, 202
    Cryotherapy, 160, 202
    Detoxification therapy, 202

Diet, 124-126, 131, 134-156 203
EMDR, 203
Energy medicine, 51, 201, 203
Environmental medicine 204
Enzyme therapy, 204
Fasting, 204
Flower remedies, 204
Guided imagery, 205
Herbal medicine, 200, 205
Homeopathy, 205-206
Hypnotherapy, 206
Juice therapy, 206
Low-Level Laser Therapy (LLLT), 206-207
Meditation. Also See
Meditations and Exercises. 21-23, 38, 43, 51, 61-62, 65, 76, 139, 148-151, 166, 171, 191, 200, 207-208.
Naturopathic medicine, 207
Narrative therapy, 207
Nutritional supplements. See also Supplements. 208
Qigong, 21, 29, 50, 74, 201, 208
Raindrop technique therapy, 159, 208
Reiki, 208
Reflexology, 209
Watsu (water shiatsu), 209
Yoga, 21-23, 41, 59, 136-138, 149-151, 197, 200, 209
Healing remedies, 147-162
    Aloe Vera, 157
    Astragalus, 157
    Baking soda, 134, 158
    Black tea, 158
    Body Balance, 157, 162

Carrageenan, 103-104, 138
Coconut oil, 160,
Colloidal silver, 157-158
Corn starch, 158
Dandelion, 158
Epson salt bath, 158
Essential oil, 158-159, 163, 200, 208, 212
Garlic, 32, 113, 135, 140, 142, 150, 154, 159, 203
Goldenseal, 159
Gum-omile, 163
Ice, 160
Holy basil/tusli, 159
Lauricidin, 157, 160, 212
Lemon balm (Melissa officinalis), 158, 160, 200, 121,
Licorice root and DGL, 160-161
Lysine, 92, 137, 142-145, 149-151 161, 164
Medicinal mushrooms, 161
Olive leaf extract, 161, 200
Pau d'arco, 162, 164
Prunella vulgaris, 161
Red clover, 162
Rescue remedy, 161
Seaweed, 103, 162
Siberian ginseng, 162
St. John's wort, 162
Taheebo, 162, 164
Vitamin E, 163
Vita-myr, 164
Heavy metals, 29, 124-127, 131-134, 141, 153, 156, 202
Herpes
    Chickenpox (Varicella Zoster), 81

Cold sores, 62, 81, 89, 92-93, 100-101, 114, 118, 120, 177-178. See also Herpes Simplex 1 (HSV-1)
Cytomegalovirus, 82
Gladiatorum, 82
Genital herpes. 20, 37, 62, 73, 80-92, 100-101, 103, 106, 114-121, 129, 137, 153, 179, 201. See also Herpes Simplex 2 (HSV-2)
Herpetic whitlow, 82
Human Herpes Virus 6, 82
Human Herpes Virus 7, 82
Human Herpes Virus 8, 82
Herpes Simplex 1 (HSV-1), 81-86, 92, 96, 98-117, 161
Herpes Simplex 2 (HSV-2), 81-91, 96-108, 116-117, 161
Kaposi's Sarcoma, 82
Mononucleosis (Mono or Epstein-Barr virus), 82, 85, 114
Neonatal herpes, 113-118, 121
Ocular herpes (Herpes Simplex Keratitis) 93
Oral-facial, 27-28, 30, 82, 89, 102, 118, 128, 152-153. See also Herpes Simplex 1 (HSV-1).
Oral herpes, 2, 163-164
Roseola, 82, 114
Shingles (Herpes Zoster), 81, 92, 114, 157, 160
Herpetic whitlow. See Herpes.
Holistic medicine, 30-34, 38, 71
Hologram, 30
Hormonal imbalance, 138, 152

Horizontal transmission, 83
HSV-I and HSV-2. See Herpes.
Ice. See Cryotherapy.
Immune system, 22, 25, 38, 82, 92-93,
    108-109, 115,120, 125, 127,
    129, 160, 202, 205, 207, 209
Infertility, 49, 128, 133, 155
Initial diagnosis, 24, 40, 113
Intuition, 27, 64-71, 170, 189
IUD, 153

Jack Canfield, 57, 184, 213
Journaling, 25, 139, 150-151, 167, 189,

Learner, 53-57
Louise Hay, 60-62

Meditations and exercises
    A List of De-stressors, 196
    Accessing Your Inner Guru, 195-196
    Affirmations, 62-62
    An Exercise of Forgiveness, 50-52
    Breath Is Life, 75-78
    Building Self Confidence, 192-193
    Call Your Power Back, 74-75
    Daily Dose, 197-198
    First Chakra Clearing, 73-74
    Elevator Exercise, 70-71
    Eliminating Your Fears Before
    Having "the Talk", 183-185
    Healing With Positive Thinking,
    59-60
    Meditation Made Simple, 191
    My Pink Diary, 189-190
    Raising The Root of Self
    Esteem, 193-194
    Rejuvenating Meditation, 191

Sushi Size Your Day, 195
    Taking The Charge Out, 181-183
Mercury, 124, 126, 128, 151-154
Milia, 121
Mineral Deficiencies, 123-126
Misdiagnoses, 99-100, 109
Mononucleosis (Mono). See Herpes.

NHANES study, 90-91
Nervous system, 23, 33, 76, 124, 134,
    154, 160-161, 163, 201-202
Newborn. See Herpes-Neonatal
Nonoxyldol-9 (N-9), 103-104

Omega 3's. See Supplements
Oral sex, 92, 109, 117
Outbreaks, 24-25, 27-34, 36-38, 46,
    82, 88, 93-94, 113, 119, 123-129,
    136-138, 142-144, 152-153,
    156-164, 170-171, 190-191

Phases of Healing, 87
Pregnancy and delivery, 113-121
    Antibodies, 115, 117, 120
    C-section, 2, 118
    Fetal monitoring, 116
Premature rupture of
    Membranes, 116
    Vaginal delivery, 2, 116, 119, 121
Prodrome, 86, 92, 104

Reactivation, 80, 84

Sacral nerves, 80-81, 153
Self care plan, 147-164
Sex toys, 83
Sexual abuse, 49-50, 61, 139, 152

Sexuality, 62, 129
Shingles. See Herpes.
STD's
    Chlamydia, 96, 111
    Genital warts, 96, 108, 112
    Gonorrhea, 109-110
    HIV, 110-112, 162, 179, 22, 33, 61, 96
    HPV, 96, 108-109, 112, 129
    Pubic lice, 111-112
    Syphilis, 110-111
    Trichomoniasis (Trich), 113
Surrender, 19, 23, 29-31, 35, 44, 47,
    167-168, 170-171
Still period, 41-44
Sunshine. See Triggers.
Supplements, 35, 38, 71, 138, 142,
    147-156, 190, 208 D3, 150, 155
    Kelp, 126, 153-156
    Lysine, 142
    Multivitamin, 143, 149-150, 155
    Omega 3's-149, 152, 154
    Probiotics, 111, 113, 135, 152,
    153, 202
    Selenium, 150, 155, 159
    Zinc, 124-127, 138, 149-150,
    152-153, 155, 164,
Symptoms. See also Herpes-neonatal,
    88-90, 93, 100-104, 106,
    108-114, 121, 136-139, 144,
    147-148, 150-151, 163, 170-
    171, 175, 178, 189, 199
Synchronicities, 65, 68-69

Telling a partner. See "the Talk".
The Talk, 28, 48, 172-185
Testing, 91, 96-100
    Culture, 97
    False negatives, 97

Polymerase Chain Reaction (PCR),
    97-98, 101
    Swab, 96-101
    Western blot test, 98
Toilet seats. See Transmission
Toxicities
    Deodorant, 128, 133
    Food, 124-128, 131-132
    Electromagnetic pollution, 129-130
    Tampons, 129
Transmission, 83, 84, 90-91, 99, 103,
    105, 107, 114, 116-120, 176, 178
    Autoinoculation, 83, 93
    Congenital transmission, 83
    Horizontal transmission, 83
    Sex toys, 83
    Toilet seats, 37
    Vertical transmission, 83
Triad of health, 29
Triggers,
    Arginine 127, 137, 138, 142-145,
    149-154, 161
    Caffeine, 25, 37, 134, 143, 159,
    196
    Chocolate, 37, 127, 137, 143,149,
    152
    Emotions, 27-28
    Journaling and triggers, 189-190
    Nightshades, 144-145
    Nuts, 154, 37, 125, 127, 137, 143,
    149,152, 157
    Sunshine, 136-137, 153
    Trauma, 139, 153
    Top 10 triggers, 156-159

Valtrex, See antivirals
Victim/Victor, 31, 36, 42-44, 54,
    57-48, 61, 180

Viral shedding. See Asymptomatic
   shedding

Western medicine, 26, 30-34
Weil, Andrew MD, 130, 160
Wilson, Lawrence MD, 29, 124,
   212-213
Wrestlers, 82

Wright, Lance DC, 24-25

Yeast infections, 88-90, 113, 135,
   143,150, 152-153
Yoga, 21-23, 41, 59, 136-138,
   149-151, 197, 200, 209

Zinc. See Supplements

Made in the USA
Lexington, KY
06 January 2015